ACID ALKALINE DIET COOKBOOK

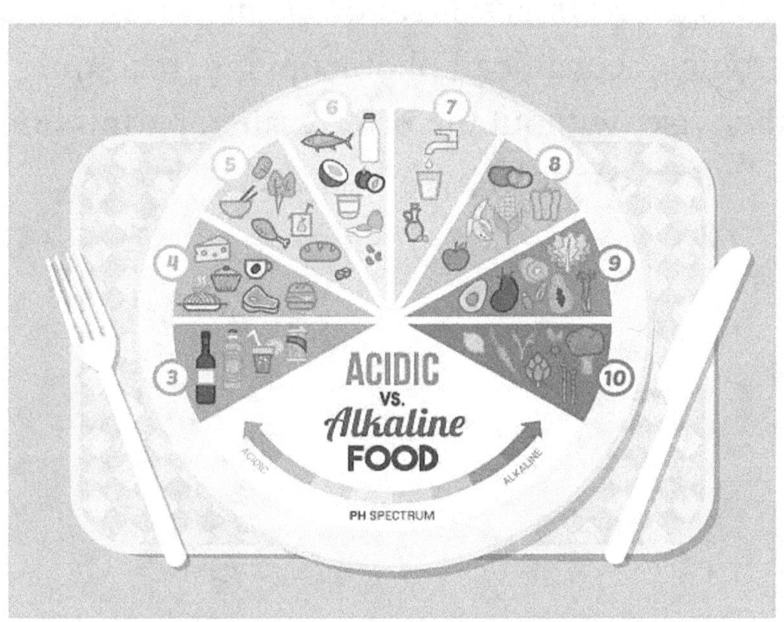

DISCOVER THE EASIEST WAY TO IMPROVE YOUR HEALTH THROUGH PH BALANCE DIET

Dr. Samuel Jackson

Copyright (c) 2023 Dr. Samuel Jackson

TABLE OF CONTENTS

INTRODUCTION

Are you tired of feeling constantly run down, struggling with inflammation and chronic health issues, and just not feeling your best? It's a frustrating and exhausting experience that can leave you feeling stuck and hopeless.

I understand the pain points that comes with feeling like your body is working against you. I know what it's like to struggle with fatigue, inflammation, and a host of other health issues that can make you feel like you're not living up to your potential.

That's why I've created an acid alkaline diet cookbook that is designed specifically to address these pain points. The recipes in this book are carefully crafted to help balance the pH levels in your body, reduce inflammation, and support optimal health and wellbeing.

I know that making changes to your diet can feel overwhelming and intimidating, which is why I've made this cookbook as approachable and easy to use as possible. The recipes are delicious, satisfying, and made with real, whole foods that will leave you feeling nourished and energized.

I believe that everyone deserves to feel their best, no matter what health issues they may be facing. That's why I've made it our mission to provide a solution that can help you take control of your health and start feeling better than ever before.

So if you're tired of feeling like your body is working against you, and you're ready to take the first step towards a healthier, happier you, then I encourage you to give our acid alkaline diet cookbook a try. You deserve to feel your best, and we're here to help you get there

Welcome to my acid alkaline diet cookbook! This book is your ultimate guide to understanding the benefits of an alkaline diet, and how to incorporate it into your daily life through delicious and nourishing recipes.

The concept of this acid alkaline diet is based on the idea that certain foods can affect the pH levels in your body. By eating a diet that is high in alkaline foods and low in acidic foods, you can help balance these levels and support optimal health and wellbeing.

This cookbook is filled with over 50 delicious and easy-to-make recipes that will help you incorporate more alkaline foods into your diet. From vibrant smoothie bowls to hearty soups and stews, you will find a variety of options for every meal of the day.

But this cookbook is more than just a collection of recipes. It's also a comprehensive guide to understanding the science behind an acid alkaline diet, and how it can help reduce inflammation, boost energy levels, and support overall health and wellbeing.

Whether you are new to the concept of an acid alkaline diet, or you are looking for new and exciting recipes to add to your repertoire, this cookbook has something for everyone. I believe that eating healthy shouldn't mean sacrificing flavor or satisfaction, and I have created recipes that are both nourishing and delicious.

So join me on this journey towards optimal health and wellbeing. Let this cookbook be your guide to a healthier, happier you!

OVERVIEW OF THE ACID ALKALINE DIET

The foundation of the acid alkaline diet—also referred to as the alkaline diet—is the idea that specific meals can either contribute to an acidic or alkaline environment in the body. Diet advocates claim that consuming a diet rich in alkaline foods and low in acidic foods can aid in balancing the pH levels of the body, which can have a number of positive health effects.

The foundation of the acid-alkaline diet is the notion that the foods we eat can directly affect the pH levels of our bodies. The pH scale, with a neutral value of 7, determines how acidic or alkaline a substance is. The pH range of the human body is naturally 7.35-7.45, which makes it somewhat alkaline. Although many of the meals we consume are acidic, this delicate equilibrium can be upset.

The idea behind the acid-alkaline diet is that by eating a diet that is high in alkaline foods and low in acidic foods, we can support optimal health and wellbeing and help to restore this equilibrium. those that are alkaline have a pH greater than 7, while those that are acidic have a pH lower than 7.

Leafy greens, cruciferous vegetables like broccoli and cauliflower, fruits like berries and melons, nuts and seeds, and certain grains like quinoa and millet are some of the most popular alkaline foods. On the other side, some of the most popular acidic foods are sugar, coffee, processed foods, meat, dairy, and dairy products.

The precise ratios of alkaline and acidic foods will vary based on an individual's demands and health objectives. The acid-alkaline diet is not a one-size-fits-all approach. While some diet advocates advocate a ratio of 80% alkaline foods to 20% acidic foods, others advocate a more moderate ratio of 60% alkaline foods to 40% acidic foods.

The acid-alkaline diet has been linked to a variety of health advantages in addition to balancing the pH levels in the body. According to some research, an alkaline diet may help to lower inflammation, strengthen bones, maintain renal function, and even lower the chance of developing chronic diseases like cancer and heart disease.

We've developed a collection of recipes for the acid alkaline diet cookbook that are intended to help you increase the amount of alkaline foods in your diet. We have you covered with tasty and wholesome meals that will help you feel your best, from smoothie bowls and salads to soups, stews, and even desserts

BENEFITS OF AN ALKALINE DIET

Alkaline diets, which are based on the idea that particular foods can either contribute to an acidic or alkaline environment in the body, are gaining popularity due to their possible health benefits. An alkaline diet may have a variety of health advantages, although additional research is need to fully understand these effects.

The following are some possible advantages of an alkaline diet:

Reduced inflammation: Anti-inflammatory substances like antioxidants are abundant in many alkaline meals, which may aid to lessen inflammation in the body. Numerous health issues, including as autoimmune illnesses, cancer, and heart disease, have been related to chronic inflammation.

An alkaline diet may assist to promote bone health by lowering the risk of osteoporosis, according to certain research. This may be because alkaline foods aid to maintain calcium levels in the bones whereas acidic foods can cause calcium to be lost from the bones.

Improved kidney function: An alkaline diet may support kidney function because the kidneys are important for controlling the body's pH levels. An alkaline diet may help to lower the risk of kidney stones and enhance overall kidney health, according to studies.

A more alkaline diet may help lower the chance of developing chronic diseases including cancer and heart disease, however more research is required in this area. This could be as a result of the fact that alkaline foods are frequently rich in minerals and antioxidants that can assist to prevent cellular damage and inflammation.

Improved digestive health: The high fiber content of many alkaline foods can assist to encourage good digestion and lower the risk of issues like constipation and bloating.

Increased energy: By lowering inflammation and giving the body the nutrition it needs to perform at its best, an alkaline diet may help to enhance energy levels.

Although an alkaline diet has some promise health advantages, it's crucial to remember that more research is required to completely comprehend its effects. Additionally, based on a person's demands and health objectives, the precise proportions of alkaline and acidic foods that are best for health may change.

I've developed a collection of recipes for the acid-alkaline diet cookbook that are intended to help you increase the amount of alkaline foods in your diet. The recipes in this book can assist

you in achieving your health objectives, whether you want to lessen inflammation, strengthen your bones, or just feel your best.

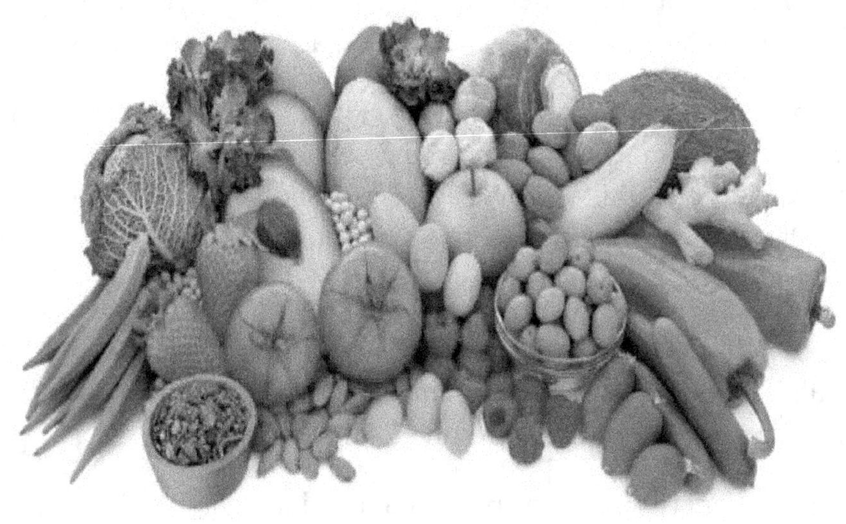

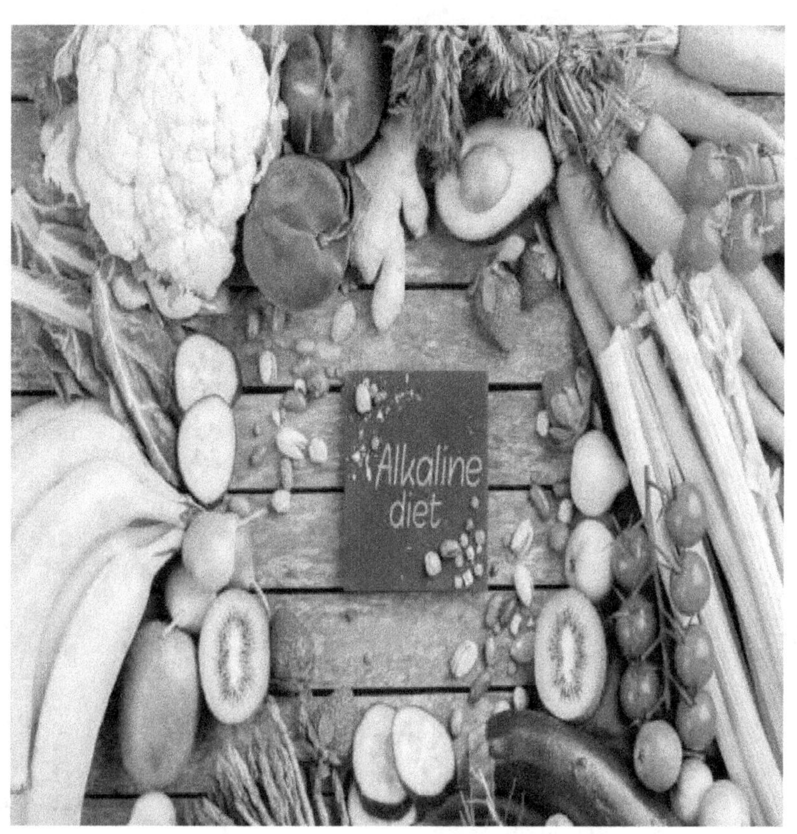

CHAPTER 1

UNDERSTANDING PH BALANCE

The term "pH balance" refers to the harmony between an object's acidity and alkalinity, and it is vital to how the human body functions. The pH scale has a range of 0 to 14, with 7 being regarded as neutral. Anything that is alkaline or basic is anything that is over 7, whereas anything that is below 7 is considered acidic.

The ideal pH for each organ and system varies within the human body. For instance, the stomach's high acidity (pH range: 1.5–3.5) aids in the breakdown of food and the eradication of dangerous microorganisms. The blood, on the other hand, has a closely controlled, slightly alkaline pH range of 7.35 to 7.45.

Too much acidity or alkalinity in the body's pH can interfere with healthy biological processes and cause a variety of health issues. For instance, the presence of acidic conditions in the body has been associated with inflammation, impaired immune response, and a higher chance of developing chronic illnesses including cancer and heart disease. Alkalosis, on the other hand, is a disorder that can result from the body becoming overly alkaline and can include symptoms including disorientation, twitching muscles, and nausea.

The pH balance of the body can be impacted by a variety of things, such as nutrition, stress, exercise, and environmental influences. Dietary choices can influence whether a person's body is more alkaline or more acidic. As an illustration, meals strong in protein like meat, dairy products, and eggs are frequently acidic while fruits, vegetables, and some grains are typically more alkaline.

Eat more alkaline foods, according to some proponents of the alkaline diet, to assist the body's pH balance and promote good health. To completely comprehend the impacts of an alkaline diet on health outcomes, more study is necessary.

The human body needs a pH balance to function properly, and imbalances can cause a variety of health issues. pH balance can be impacted by a variety of things, including nutrition, stress, and exercise. You can use the recipes in our cookbook for the acid-alkaline diet to add more alkaline foods to your diet and support optimum health.

Ph Balance: A Science

Acid-base chemistry, which examines how acids and bases behave in aqueous solutions, is the foundation of the science of pH balance. The quantity of hydrogen ions ($H+$) in the solution determines pH, which is a measure of a substance's acidity or alkalinity.

The pH scale has a range of 0 to 14, with 7 being regarded as neutral. Anything that is alkaline or basic is anything that is over 7, whereas anything that is below 7 is considered acidic. Since the pH scale is logarithmic, a change of one unit corresponds to a tenfold increase or decrease in acidity or alkalinity. For instance, a pH of 5 solution is ten times more acidic than a pH of 6 solution.

Numerous processes in the human body need precise pH management to work properly. For instance, blood pH must be kept within the specific range of 7.35 to 7.45 to guarantee optimal oxygen delivery, enzyme activity, and other crucial processes. Depending on whether the blood's pH is too low or too high, when it is outside of this range, it can cause a condition known as acidosis or alkalosis.

The kidneys, lungs, and buffer systems are only a few of the body's many regulatory systems that control pH equilibrium. The lungs assist in regulating the quantity of carbon dioxide in the body, which can impact blood pH, while the kidneys assist in eliminating extra acids or bases from the body. By binding or releasing hydrogen ions, buffer systems, which include substances like bicarbonate, phosphate, and proteins, can aid in the resistance to pH shifts.

The pH balance of the body can also be impacted by diet. Certain meals can contribute to an acidic or alkaline environment in the body, even if their own pH does not always directly correlate with how they affect the pH of the body. Protein-rich foods like meat, dairy, and eggs are frequently acidic, whereas fruits, vegetables, and some grains are typically more alkaline.

Eat more alkaline foods, according to some proponents of the alkaline diet, to assist the body's pH balance and promote good health. However, additional research is required to completely comprehend the intricate interactions between nutrition, pH balance, and health consequences. Research on the impacts of diet on pH balance and overall health is still in its early stages.

The science of pH balance, which involves numerous systems and methods to control the acidity and alkalinity of the body's fluids, is a complicated and crucial part of human physiology. In addition to diet, stress, exercise, and medical problems can all have an impact on pH levels. More research is necessary to completely grasp the consequences for health.

PH BALANCE AND THE BODY

The balance of acid and alkaline compounds in bodily fluids such blood, urine, and saliva is referred to as pH balance. Since many of the body's vital processes and activities depend on a certain pH range, maintaining a healthy pH balance is crucial for achieving optimal health.

The pH range of the human body is between 7.35 and 7.45, making it somewhat alkaline. A number of processes, including the kidneys, lungs, and buffer systems, work together to closely manage this range. The lungs assist in regulating carbon dioxide levels, which can impact blood pH, while the kidneys are in charge of excreting extra acids or bases from the body. By binding or releasing hydrogen ions, buffer systems, which are made up of substances like bicarbonate, phosphate, and proteins, help to resist pH shifts.

Too acidic or alkaline a pH in the body can disturb normal cellular functions and result in health issues. For instance, the condition known as acidosis, which manifests as disorientation, sluggishness, and coma, can happen when the blood pH drops below 7.35. Muscle twitching, nausea, and convulsions are just a few of the symptoms that can result from alkalosis, which happens when blood pH rises above 7.45.

The pH balance of the body can be impacted by a number of things, including nutrition, stress, activity, and medical problems. A diet rich in acidic foods, such as meat, dairy, and processed meals, can, for instance, contribute to the body's acidic environment. By raising the body's production of stress hormones, which can increase acid production, prolonged stress and sleep deprivation can also cause acidosis.

A diet high in alkaline foods, on the other hand, like fruits, vegetables, and some grains, can support the body's natural tendency toward a more alkaline environment. By enhancing circulation and oxygenation, regular exercise can also help lower acid levels in the body.

For optimum health and welfare, a balanced pH balance must be maintained. Although the body has several ways to control pH levels, other elements including nutrition, stress, and exercise can also have an impact. People can maintain their body's pH balance, advance general health and wellbeing, and support their lifestyle choices by eating a balanced diet.

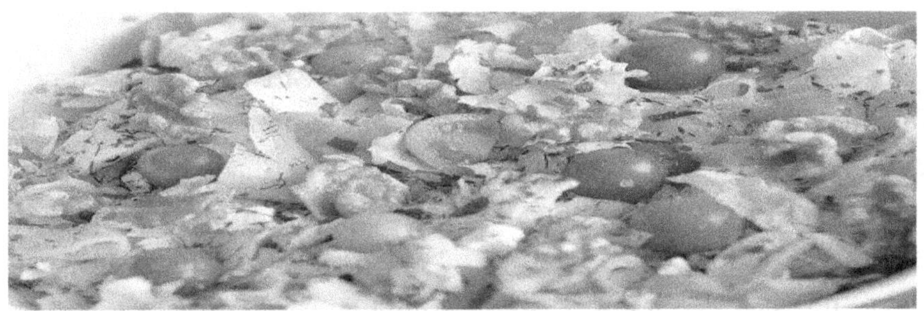

CHAPTER 2

THE ACID-ALKALINE FOOD CHART

The acid-alkaline food chart is a tool that enables people to comprehend how different foods affect the pH balance of the body and their pH values. Based on their pH level, the chart classifies foods as acidic, neutral, or alkaline. those that are acidic have a pH level below 7, while those that are alkaline have a pH level over 7. Foods that are neutral have a pH of 7. Common foods and drinks are often listed on the chart along with their matching pH value and category.

The concept behind the acid-alkaline food chart is that eating too many acidic foods might result in an imbalance in the pH of the body, which can have negative health effects. For instance, eating a lot of acidic meals can increase your risk of kidney stones, osteoporosis, and acid reflux. A diet high in alkaline foods, on the other hand, may help to encourage a more alkaline environment in the body and lower the risk of certain health problems. Typically made from plants, alkaline foods include fruits, vegetables, nuts, seeds, and some grains.

The pH value of foods is not the only thing that impacts the body's pH equilibrium, despite the fact that the acid-alkaline food chart can be a useful tool. Other elements can also come into play, including stress, physical activity, and health issues. It's also crucial to keep in mind that not all foods, whether they are alkaline or acidic, are healthy. Citrus fruits like lemons and oranges, for instance, are acidic but also packed with nutrients that are vital for good health.

For those who want to improve their diets and maintain the pH balance of their bodies, the acid-alkaline food chart might be a helpful resource. Individuals may be able to encourage optimum health and wellness by increasing their intake of alkaline foods and decreasing their consumption of acidic foods.

The pH Scale

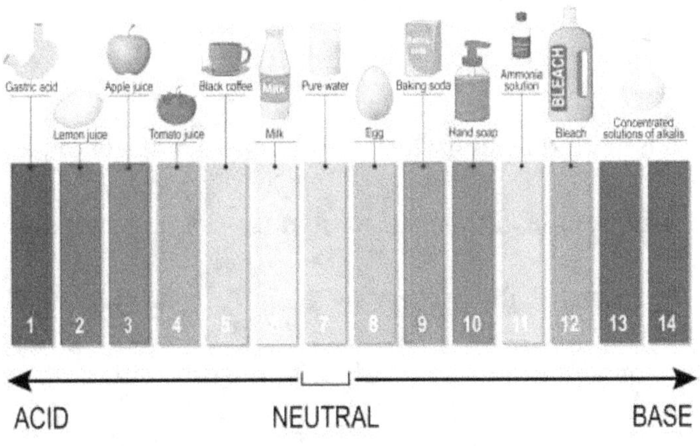

EATING AN ALKALINE DIET

An alkaline diet includes foods that promote an acidic rather than an alkaline environment in the body. This approach of eating is based on the idea that an excessively acidic diet can lead to a variety of health issues, such as inflammation, digestive problems, and a higher risk of developing chronic illnesses. By consuming more alkaline foods, people can promote their bodies' enhanced pH balance and general wellness.

Alkaline foods include things like raw fruits and vegetables, nuts, seeds, lentils, and some grains. Antioxidants, vitamins, and minerals, which are all essential for preserving overall health and wellness, are typically abundant in these meals. Contrarily, acidic foods such as processed meals, meats, dairy products, and refined sweets can lead to inflammation and other health issues.

One of the key benefits of an alkaline diet is its potential to reduce inflammation in the body. Chronic inflammation has been linked to several diseases, such as cancer, autoimmune diseases, and heart disease. Eating more alkaline meals and fewer acidic ones may help people reduce inflammation and their chances of developing chronic diseases.

An additional benefit of an alkaline diet is the potential to maintain a healthy digestive tract. A diet high in alkalinity may help to promote the growth of healthy gut flora, which are essential for optimal digestion and nutrient absorption. Alkaline diets' high fiber content can also help to promote regular bowel motions and ward off constipation.

Increasing your intake of alkaline foods can help you keep a healthy weight. Many alkaline foods are low in calories and high in fiber, which can help to promote fullness and discourage overeating. An alkaline diet may help promote a healthy metabolism and a decreased risk of insulin resistance and other metabolic illnesses.

To increase the amount of alkaline foods in your diet, concentrate on consuming a variety of fresh fruits and vegetables, such as leafy greens, cruciferous vegetables, and citrus fruits. Nuts, seeds, and legumes such as beans and lentils are also rich sources of alkaline elements. Avoid processed and refined foods, as well as meat and dairy products, which might result in an excessively acidic diet.

An excellent way to support healthy weight management and advance optimal health is by following an alkaline diet. By eating more alkaline foods and fewer acidic ones, you can help your body maintain a healthier pH balance and reduce your chance of developing chronic diseases.

FOODS TO EAT AND AVOID FOR A ACID ALKALINE DIET

The premise of the acid-alkaline diet is that eating foods that are more alkaline than acidic would improve your health and that certain meals can alter the pH balance in your body. The following foods should be included in an acid-alkaline diet and should be avoided:

FOOD TO EAT

Vegetables: The majority of vegetables, especially leafy greens like spinach, kale, and collard greens, as well as cruciferous veggies like broccoli, cauliflower, and Brussels sprouts, are alkaline-forming.

Fruits: Most fruits are alkaline-forming, especially citrus fruits like lemons, limes, and grapefruits as well as berries, melons, and pears.

Whole grains: Quinoa, brown rice, and whole wheat bread are examples of whole grains that can produce alkali.

Nuts and seeds that produce alkalinity include almonds, sunflower seeds, and pumpkin seeds.

Plant-based protein: Legumes like lentils, chickpeas, and black beans, as well as tofu and tempeh, are alkaline-forming sources of protein.

FOOD TO AVOID

Fast food, snack meals, and beverages with added sugar are all examples of excessively processed foods that are quite acidic.

Animal protein: Meat, fish, poultry, and dairy products are examples of acidic foods.

White bread, spaghetti, and other refined grains are among the acidic foods.

Fried foods, fatty meat cuts, and full-fat dairy products are examples of acidic foods.

Artificial sweeteners: Two examples of artificial sweeteners that are acidic are aspartame and saccharin.

You don't need to perfectly follow an acid-alkaline diet to stay healthy; while some foods may be more alkaline-forming or acidic than others, your body has a built-in system for maintaining a good pH balance. The classification of foods as "acidic" or "alkaline" is not always straightforward because some acidic meals, such citrus fruits, can also have alkaline effects on the body after digestion.

The acid-alkaline diet has not been proven scientifically, but it can be a helpful way to focus on consuming more filling, nutrient-dense foods that are beneficial for overall health. If you focus on a plant-based diet, you'll inadvertently consume more fiber, vitamins, and minerals that are essential for optimum health.

Along with the above-mentioned meals to consume and steer clear of, it's important to pay attention to portion sizes and eat a variety of foods. By consuming a variety of plant-based foods, you can make sure that your body is receiving all the nutrients it needs. Another wise choice is to consume enough of water, which can support your body's natural pH balance.

Although the acid-alkaline diet may not be a miracle cure, it can offer a helpful framework for making better dietary choices. But it's important to remember that everyone has unique nutritional requirements, so what suits one person may not suit another. If you have any concerns about your diet or health, it's always a good idea to speak with a qualified healthcare practitioner.

TIPS FOR MEAL PLANNING AND GROCERY SHOPPING

Here are some tips for meal planning and grocery shopping for an acid alkaline diet:

Focus Your Menus On Plant-Based Items.

Give meals that feature a range of fruits, vegetables, whole grains, legumes, nuts, and seeds special attention. These foods offer a plethora of nutrients that are crucial for good health and are typically alkaline-forming.

Alkaline And Acidic Foods In Moderation

While eating more alkaline-forming foods is crucial, you need also balance them with acidic meals to make sure your body is getting all the nutrients it needs. For instance, combine alkaline-producing greens like spinach or kale with acidic meals like tomatoes or vinegar.

Be Mindful Of Portion Sizes

It is possible to upset your body's natural pH balance by consuming too much of any one item, even an alkaline-forming food. Consider your portion amounts and try to include a variety of meals at each meal.

Select Unprocessed, Whole Foods

Processed meals, even those promoted as "healthy" or "natural," frequently have extra sugars, bad fats, and other ingredients that might be toxic for your body. As much as possible, stick to complete, unadulterated foods.

View Labels

When purchasing packaged foods, pay close attention to the ingredients list. Eat less food that has artificial sweeteners, extra sugars, or other unhealthy ingredients.

Shop Outside The Store

Most grocery stores often have whole grains, fresh fruits and vegetables, and other whole foods around the outside of the store. Instead of concentrating your buying efforts in the center aisles, which typically include more processed items, do so here.

Bulk Purchases

Bulk purchases of grains, nuts, and seeds can be an economical way to stock up on wholesome essentials.

Take In A Lot Of Water

Water consumption can support the pH balance that your body naturally maintains. In order to stay hydrated during the day, carry a reusable water bottle with you.

Try Out Different Recipes

Meal planning can be made more exciting and fun by experimenting with different recipes. Look for meals that use alkaline-forming foods like cruciferous vegetables, leafy greens, and plant-based meats.

Prepare Meals In Advance

Making a weekly meal plan will help you make sure you eat a variety of foods and receive all the nutrients you need. Set aside some time each week to compile a grocery list and plan your meals.

Do Not Be Frightened To Experiment

Eating a balanced, healthy diet doesn't have to be monotonous. To keep things exciting and delightful, experiment with new cuisines, flavors, and cooking techniques.

Utilize Spices And Herbs

Spices and herbs are excellent ways to flavor your food without increasing the acidity. Try out several herbs and spices to find flavor combinations you like.

Pay Attention To Food Sensitivities

Consider any food allergies or sensitivities you may have when making meal plans and grocery shopping. Look for substitute items that you can ingest.

Think About Taking Supplements

While whole meals are the finest source of nutrients, some people may benefit from taking supplements to support their body's natural pH balance. Consult a licensed healthcare professional to determine whether supplements is appropriate for you.

Keep in mind that everyone has different nutritional needs and that the acid-alkaline diet is only one method of a balanced diet. You may design a healthy, balanced diet that works for you by emphasizing whole, unprocessed foods and a range of various fruits, vegetables, whole grains, legumes, nuts, and seeds.

ALKALINE REPLACEMENTS FOR

TYPICAL ACIDIC FOODS

A wonderful strategy to change your diet to have a more alkaline balance is to replace typical acidic meals with alkaline alternatives. You can replace the following foods in your diet to make it more alkaline by:

Use almond milk in place of dairy milk: Almond milk is alkaline whereas dairy milk is acidic. A good source of calcium, vitamin D, and other minerals is almond milk.

Replace white bread with whole grain bread because white bread, which is created from refined flour, is acidic, while whole grain bread, which is made from whole grains rich in fiber and other nutrients, is alkaline.

Use coconut aminos instead of soy sauce because they are alkaline instead of acidic. Coconut aminos are created from coconut tree sap and have less salt than soy sauce, yet they have a flavor that is similar to soy sauce.

Replace coffee with herbal tea instead of coffee because herbal tea is alkaline and can hydrate while coffee is acidic and can dehydrate. Several health advantages can be obtained from drinking herbal teas like peppermint, chamomile, and ginger.

Use lemon juice instead of vinegar: Lemon juice is alkaline-forming in the body, whereas vinegar is acidic. In salad dressings and other dishes, it can be substituted for vinegar.

Use avocado instead of mayonnaise since it is alkaline and a good source of healthy fats while mayonnaise is acidic and heavy in bad fats. Mayonnaise can be substituted with mashed avocado in sandwiches and salads.

Replace red meat with plant-based proteins: While plant-based proteins like tofu, tempeh, and beans are alkaline and sometimes high in fiber and other nutrients, red meat is acidic and can be high in saturated fats.

You may assist your body in moving toward a more alkaline balance by incorporating these and other alkaline replacements into your diet. To make sure you're getting all the nutrients your body requires, keep an eye out for whole, unprocessed foods and consume a range of various fruits, vegetables, whole grains, legumes, nuts, and seeds.

CHAPTER 3

RECIPES FOR ALKALINE BREAKFASTS

Alkaline breakfasts are a great way to start your day off on the right foot. These breakfasts are designed to be high in alkalizing foods, which can help balance your body's pH levels and promote overall health.

When creating smoothies and juices for an acid-alkaline diet, it is important to keep the following tips in mind:

- Use mostly alkaline fruits and vegetables, such as leafy greens, cucumbers, celery, avocados, and berries.

- Use acidic fruits and vegetables in moderation, such as citrus fruits, pineapples, and tomatoes.

- Use unsweetened almond milk, coconut milk, or other plant-based milks instead of dairy milk.

- Use herbs and spices, like ginger and mint, to add flavor and alkalinity to your drinks.

- Avoid adding sweeteners, like sugar or honey, as they can be highly acidic.

By following these tips, you can create delicious and healthy smoothies and juices that will help to balance the pH levels in your body.

Here are some delicious and nutritious alkaline breakfast recipes that you can try at home.

Green Smoothie Bowl

Ingredients

1 banana

1 cup frozen spinach

1/2 cup frozen mango chunks

1/2 avocado

1/2 cup unsweetened almond milk

1/4 cup fresh mint leaves

1 tbsp chia seeds

1 tbsp hemp seeds

1 tbsp honey

Instructions

- Add all the ingredients to a blender and blend until smooth.

- Pour the smoothie into a bowl and sprinkle with additional chia seeds and hemp seeds.

- Serve and enjoy!

Prep Time: 5 minutes

Quinoa Breakfast Bowl

Ingredients

1/2 cup cooked quinoa

1/2 avocado, diced

1/2 cup cherry tomatoes, halved

1/4 cup chopped fresh cilantro

1/4 cup chopped red onion

1/4 cup cooked black beans

Juice of 1/2 lime

Salt and pepper to taste

Instructions

- In a bowl, mix together the quinoa, avocado, cherry tomatoes, cilantro, red onion, and black beans.

- Squeeze lime juice over the top and season with salt and pepper.

- Serve and enjoy!

Prep Time: 10 minutes

Alkaline Pancakes

Ingredients

1 cup almond flour

1/4 cup coconut flour

1/4 cup flaxseed meal

2 tsp baking powder

1/2 tsp sea salt

1 cup unsweetened almond milk

2 eggs

2 tbsp honey

1 tsp vanilla extract

Instructions

- In a bowl, mix together the almond flour, coconut flour, flaxseed meal, baking powder, and sea salt.

- In another bowl, whisk together the almond milk, eggs, honey, and vanilla extract.

- Add the wet ingredients to the dry ingredients and stir until well combined.

- Heat a non-stick pan over medium heat.

- Scoop about 1/4 cup of the batter onto the pan for each pancake.

- Cook for 2-3 minutes on each side or until golden brown.

- Serve with fresh berries and almond butter.

Prep Time: 15 minutes

Avocado Toast with Smoked Salmon

Ingredients

2 slices of sprouted grain bread

1 avocado, mashed

Juice of 1/2 lemon

Salt and pepper to taste

2 oz smoked salmon

1 tbsp capers

1 tbsp chopped fresh dill

Instructions

- Toast the bread.

- In a bowl, mix together the mashed avocado, lemon juice, salt, and pepper.

- Spread the avocado mixture onto the toast.

- Top each slice with smoked salmon, capers, and fresh dill.

- Serve and enjoy!

Prep Time: 10 minutes

Chia Seed Pudding

Ingredients

1/4 cup chia seeds

1 cup unsweetened almond milk

1 tbsp honey

1/2 tsp vanilla extract

Fresh berries for topping

Instructions

- In a bowl, whisk together the chia seeds, almond milk, honey, and vanilla extract.

Smoothies and Juices

Smoothies and juices are great additions to an acid-alkaline diet. These refreshing drinks not only provide hydration and nourishment but also help to balance the pH levels of the body. In this acid-alkaline diet cookbook, we will explore some delicious smoothie and juice recipes that will help you maintain a healthy pH balance.

Green Smoothie

Ingredients

1 banana

1 cup spinach

1/2 cup kale

1/2 cucumber

1/2 lime, juiced

1 cup unsweetened almond milk

Instruction

- Add all the ingredients to a blender.

- Blend until smooth.

- Serve immediately.

This green smoothie is an excellent way to start your day. The alkaline greens, cucumber, and lime help to balance the acidic banana, resulting in a delicious and healthy smoothie.

Berry Blast Smoothie

Ingredients

1/2 cup blueberries

1/2 cup strawberries

1 banana

1/2 lemon, juiced

1 cup unsweetened almond milk

Instructions

- Add all the ingredients to a blender.

- Blend until smooth.

- Serve immediately.

- This berry blast smoothie is loaded with antioxidants and is a great way to satisfy your sweet tooth while maintaining a healthy pH balance.

Carrot Juice

Ingredients

4 carrots, peeled and chopped

1/2 lemon, juiced

1-inch piece of ginger, peeled

1 cup water

Instructions

- Add all the ingredients to a blender.

- Blend until smooth.

- Strain the juice through a fine-mesh sieve or a nut milk bag.

- Serve immediately.

This carrot juice is not only delicious but also alkalizing. The carrots and lemon help to balance the acidic ginger, resulting in a refreshing and healthy juice.

Pineapple Ginger Juice

Ingredients

1 cup pineapple, chopped

1-inch piece of ginger, peeled

1/2 lime, juiced

1 cup water

Instructions

- Add all the ingredients to a blender.

- Blend until smooth.

- Strain the juice through a fine-mesh sieve or a nut milk bag.

- Serve immediately.

This pineapple ginger juice is a great way to boost your immune system and reduce inflammation. The alkalizing effect of the pineapple and lime help to balance the acidic ginger, resulting in a delicious and healthy juice.

Cucumber Mint Juice

Ingredients

1 cucumber, chopped

1/4 cup fresh mint leaves

1/2 lemon, juiced

1 cup water

Instructions

- Add all the ingredients to a blender.

- Blend until smooth.

- Strain the juice through a fine-mesh sieve or a nut milk bag.

- Serve immediately.

This cucumber mint juice is not only refreshing but also alkalizing. The cucumber and lemon help to balance the acidic mint, resulting in a healthy and delicious juice.

Berry and Kale Smoothie

Combine 1 cup of kale, 1/2 cup of blueberries, 1/2 cup of strawberries, 1 banana, and 1 cup of unsweetened almond milk in a blender. Blend until smooth and enjoy!

Citrus and Ginger Juice

Combine 2 oranges, 1 grapefruit, 1-inch piece of ginger, and 1 cup of water in a blender. Blend until smooth, strain the juice through a fine-mesh sieve or a nut milk bag, and enjoy!

Pineapple and Cucumber Smoothie

Combine 1 cup of pineapple, 1/2 cucumber, 1/2 lime, and 1 cup of unsweetened almond milk in a blender. Blend until smooth and enjoy!

Beet and Carrot Juice

Combine 2 beets, 4 carrots, 1/2 lemon, and 1 cup of water in a blender. Blend until smooth, strain the juice through a fine-mesh sieve or a nut milk bag, and enjoy!

One of the easiest ways to incorporate more alkalizing foods into your diet is through smoothies and juices. Not only are they a great way to get in more fruits and vegetables, but they are also a quick and easy way to prepare a healthy and nutritious meal or snack.

Incorporating smoothies and juices into your diet can be a great way to promote an acid-alkaline balance in your body. By using mostly alkaline fruits and vegetables, unsweetened plant-based milks, and avoiding sweeteners, you can create delicious and healthy drinks that will help you feel your best. Experiment with different fruits, vegetables, and herbs to find the perfect combination for you.

Oatmeal and porridge bowls

Oatmeal and porridge bowls are a popular breakfast option that can be easily incorporated into an acid alkaline diet. This type of diet is based on the idea that the pH level of the body can affect overall health, and that consuming alkaline foods can help balance the body's pH levels and prevent disease.

Oatmeal is a nutritious and filling breakfast option that is naturally low in acidity. It is made from whole grain oats, which are a good source of fiber, protein, and various vitamins and minerals. When combined with alkaline foods, such as fruits and nuts, oatmeal can be a great choice for those following an acid alkaline diet.

To make an alkaline oatmeal bowl, start by cooking a serving of oatmeal according to package instructions. Then, add in alkaline fruits such as bananas, berries, or apples. These fruits are not only alkaline, but also high in fiber and antioxidants, which can help boost overall health. Additionally, adding nuts, such as almonds or walnuts, can provide healthy fats and protein to the meal.

Another option for an alkaline breakfast bowl is to make a porridge using grains such as quinoa, amaranth, or millet. These grains are naturally alkaline and can be cooked with alkaline liquids such as coconut milk or almond milk. To add flavor and nutrition, mix in alkaline fruits like blueberries or mango, and top with nuts and seeds such as chia or pumpkin seeds.

When preparing oatmeal and porridge bowls for an acid alkaline diet, it's important to keep in mind the pH levels of the ingredients used. While oatmeal and many fruits are naturally alkaline, some ingredients such as dairy products and processed foods can be acidic and should be avoided. Additionally, cooking methods such as frying and grilling can increase the acidity of foods, so it's best to stick to steaming, boiling, or baking when possible.

Here are some additional tips and ideas for creating oatmeal and porridge bowls for an acid alkaline diet:

Use whole grains: Choose whole grain oats, quinoa, amaranth, or millet for your porridge bowls. These grains are naturally alkaline and provide a good source of fiber, protein, and nutrients.

Add alkaline fruits: Incorporate fruits that are high in alkaline such as bananas, berries, apples, or melons. These fruits are also high in antioxidants and can help reduce inflammation in the body.

Top with nuts and seeds: Nuts and seeds such as almonds, walnuts, chia, or pumpkin seeds are rich in healthy fats, protein, and minerals. They are also alkaline and can add a nice crunch and texture to your oatmeal or porridge bowl.

Use alkaline liquids: Avoid using cow's milk or other dairy products, which can be acidic. Instead, use alkaline liquids such as coconut milk, almond milk, or hemp milk to cook your grains and add to your bowl.

Add spices: Spices such as cinnamon, turmeric, or ginger are not only alkaline but also provide anti-inflammatory and immune-boosting benefits.

Avoid processed foods: Processed foods such as sugary cereals or instant oatmeal packets can be high in acidity and should be avoided. Stick to whole foods and cook your own grains and oats from scratch.

Experiment with flavors: Don't be afraid to mix and match different fruits, nuts, and spices to create unique and flavorful oatmeal and porridge bowls.

Consider food combining: Food combining is a concept in the acid alkaline diet that suggests combining foods that are similar in pH level. For example, you could pair alkaline fruits with alkaline nuts and seeds, or pair acidic fruits like oranges with acidic nuts like pecans.

By incorporating these tips into your oatmeal and porridge bowls, you can create a healthy and balanced breakfast that is both delicious and alkaline-friendly.

Egg and tofu dishes

Egg and tofu dishes can be a great source of protein and nutrition for those following an acid alkaline diet. The key to creating an alkaline-friendly egg or tofu dish is to pair it with alkaline vegetables, herbs, and spices.

Here's a detailed guide to creating egg and tofu dishes for an acid alkaline diet.

Egg Dishes

Eggs are a versatile and nutrient-dense food that can be prepared in many different ways. They are a good source of protein, vitamins, and minerals, but can be high in cholesterol, so it's important to consume them in moderation. To make an egg dish that is alkaline-friendly, consider these tips:

Use alkaline vegetables: Add alkaline vegetables such as leafy greens, broccoli, asparagus, or peppers to your egg dishes. These vegetables are high in fiber and provide vitamins and minerals that can help balance your pH levels.

Avoid dairy products: While cheese and milk are often used in egg dishes, they can be high in acidity. Instead, use non-dairy alternatives such as almond milk or coconut milk.

Use alkaline spices: Add alkaline spices such as turmeric, cumin, or coriander to your egg dishes. These spices not only add flavor but also provide anti-inflammatory and immune-boosting benefits.

Try different cooking methods: While fried eggs are a popular option, they can be high in acidity. Try steaming or poaching your eggs instead.

Pair with alkaline sides: Pair your egg dishes with alkaline sides such as roasted sweet potatoes, quinoa, or a salad made with alkaline vegetables.

Tofu Dishes

Tofu is a great source of plant-based protein and is naturally alkaline. It is made from soybeans and is rich in nutrients such as calcium, iron, and magnesium. To make an alkaline-friendly tofu dish, consider these tips:

Use alkaline vegetables: Add alkaline vegetables such as bok choy, kale, or spinach to your tofu dishes. These vegetables are high in fiber and provide vitamins and minerals that can help balance your pH levels.

Avoid processed tofu products: Tofu products such as fried tofu or flavored tofu can be high in acidity. Stick to plain, organic tofu to keep your dish alkaline.

Use alkaline spices: Add alkaline spices such as ginger, garlic, or lemongrass to your tofu dishes. These spices not only add flavor but also provide anti-inflammatory and immune-boosting benefits.

Try different cooking methods: While fried tofu is a popular option, it can be high in acidity. Try baking or grilling your tofu instead.

Pair with alkaline sides: Pair your tofu dishes with alkaline sides such as quinoa, brown rice, or a salad made with alkaline vegetables.

Egg and tofu dishes can be a healthy and satisfying option for those following an acid alkaline diet. By pairing these protein sources with alkaline vegetables, herbs, and spices, you can create a meal that is both delicious and alkaline-friendly.

Here are some additional tips and ideas for creating egg and tofu dishes for an acid alkaline diet:

Add alkaline fruits: Incorporate fruits that are high in alkaline such as avocados, tomatoes, or bell peppers into your egg or tofu dishes. These fruits are also high in antioxidants and can help reduce inflammation in the body.

Use alkaline oils: Avoid using vegetable oil or other cooking oils that can be acidic. Instead, use alkaline oils such as olive oil, coconut oil, or avocado oil to cook your eggs or tofu.

Experiment with flavors: Don't be afraid to mix and match different herbs and spices to create unique and flavorful egg and tofu dishes.

Avoid processed foods: Processed foods such as packaged tofu products or pre-made egg dishes can be high in acidity and should be avoided. Stick to whole foods and cook your own meals from scratch.

Consider food combining: Food combining is a concept in the acid alkaline diet that suggests combining foods that are similar in pH level. For example, you could pair alkaline tofu with alkaline vegetables like broccoli or asparagus.

Incorporate fermented foods: Fermented foods such as kimchi, sauerkraut, or miso can help promote healthy gut bacteria and have an alkalizing effect on the body. Consider adding these foods to your egg or tofu dishes for an extra boost of nutrition.

By incorporating these tips into your egg and tofu dishes, you can create a variety of healthy and alkaline-friendly meals that are both delicious and nutritious.

When it comes to an acid-alkaline diet, it is important to maintain a balance between alkalizing and acidic foods. While some foods, like meat, dairy, and processed foods, are considered acidic, others, like leafy greens, vegetables, and fruits, are considered alkaline. By incorporating more alkalizing foods into your diet, you can help to balance the acidity in your body and promote overall health and wellbeing.

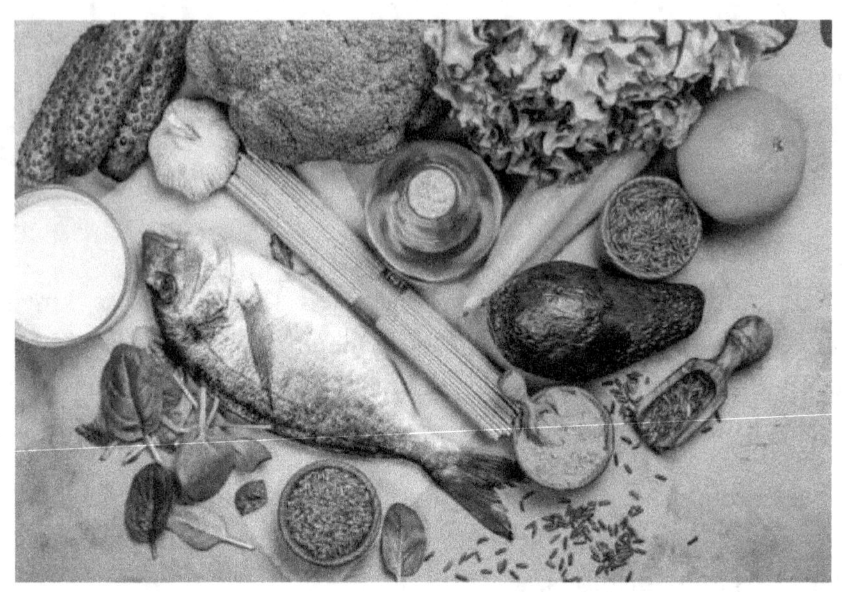

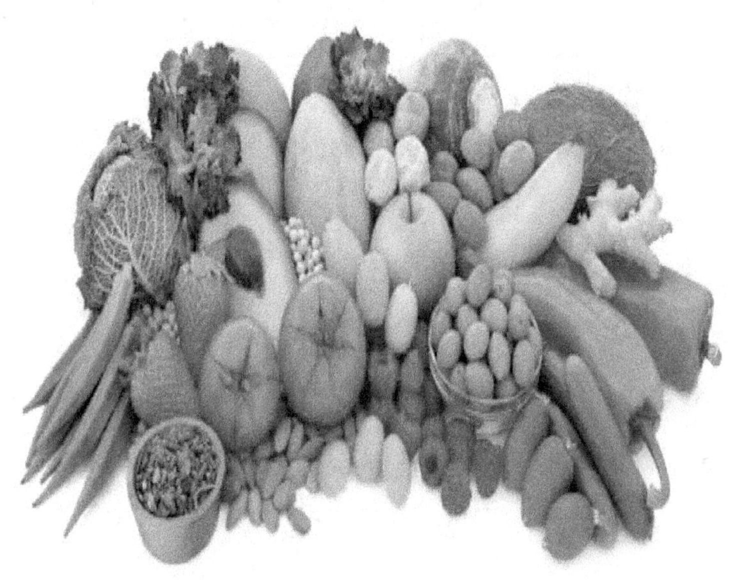

CHAPTER 4

RECIPES FOR ALKALINE LUNCH

Lentil and Vegetable Soup

Ingredients

1 cup green lentils

4 cups vegetable stock 1 diced onion

2 chopped carrots, 2 diced celery stalks

1 chopped red bell pepper

2 minced garlic cloves

1 tablespoon of olive oil

1.5 tbsp tomato paste

1 teaspoon cumin, ground

Dry thyme, 1 teaspoon

pepper and salt as desired

Instructions

Lentils should be rinsed in cold water before being added to a pot with 4 cups of vegetable broth. Bring to a boil, then lower the heat and simmer the lentils for 20 to 25 minutes, or until they are tender.

Olive oil should be heated over medium heat in a different saucepan. Add the diced red bell pepper, carrots, celery, and onion. Cook the vegetables for 5-7 minutes with occasional stirring until they are tender.

• Stir in the tomato paste, cumin, and thyme to the pot of ingredients. To blend, stir.

• Fill the pot with the cooked lentils and the broth. After combining, simmer for an additional 5 to 10 minutes.

Add salt and pepper to taste when seasoning.

Grilled chicken and a salad of vegetables

Ingredients

Sliced and grilled one chicken breast

4 cups of greens, mixed

1 cup halved cherry tomatoes

Sliced cucumber, one

14 cup of red onion slices

14 cup of almond slices

2/TBS of olive oil

Balsamic vinegar, 1 tablespoon

pepper and salt as desired

Instructions

• Heat a grill or grill pan to a moderately high temperature. Cook the chicken breast on the grill until done, then cut into strips.

• Combine the mixed greens, cherry tomatoes, cucumber slices, and red onion slices in a sizable mixing dish.

• Fill the bowl with the chicken slices.

• Combine the olive oil and balsamic vinegar thoroughly in a separate small bowl.

• Drizzle the salad with the dressing and toss to combine.

• Sprinkle sliced almonds on top of the salad and season with salt and pepper to taste.

Ingredients for the Roasted Vegetable Wrap: 1 red bell pepper, cut; 1 zucchini; 1 yellow squash; 1/4 red onion; 2 minced garlic cloves; 2 tablespoons of olive oil.

pepper and salt as desired

2 significant collard-green leaves

Instructions

Preheat the oven to 400°F. Mix the olive oil, salt, and pepper with the minced garlic and vegetable slices. Spread out on a baking sheet, then roast for 20 to 25 minutes, or until tender and just burnt.

The roasted veggies should be divided between the two collard green leaves after they have been spread out.

To form a wrap, fold the collard green leaves over the filling.

Chickpea and Avocado Salad

Ingredients

1 can of washed and drained chickpeas

1 diced avocado

1 cup halved cherry tomatoes

1/4 cup red onion, chopped

2 tbsp freshly chopped cilantro

2/TBS of olive oil

Apple cider vinegar, 1 tablespoon

pepper and salt as desired

Instructions

• Combine the chickpeas, diced avocado, cherry tomatoes, red onion, and cilantro in a sizable mixing bowl.

• Olive oil and apple cider vinegar should be thoroughly mixed in a separate small basin.

• Mix the salad thoroughly after adding the dressing.

• To taste, add salt and pepper to the food.

Stir-fried vegetables with tofu

Ingredients

1 brick of firm tofu, chopped after draining

2 cups of chopped mixed veggies, including carrots, broccoli, bell peppers, and snap peas

1 tablespoon of olive oil

2 minced garlic cloves

1-tablespoon grated ginger

2 tbsp. soy sauce

1-tablespoon rice vinegar

1 teaspoon of honey

Instructions

• In a sizable skillet or wok, heat the olive oil over medium-high heat.

• Stir-fry the tofu in diced form for 5 to 7 minutes, or until just faintly browned.

• Stir-fry the vegetables until tender-crisp for an additional 5-7 minutes after adding them to the skillet.

• Stir-fry the grated ginger and minced garlic in the skillet for an additional one to two minutes, or until fragrant.

• In a different small bowl, thoroughly blend the soy sauce, rice vinegar, and honey.

Stir-fry

Ingredients

a bowl of vegetables and quinoa

cooked quinoa, 1 cup

2 cups of greens, mixed

Half a cup of cherry tomatoes

1/4 cup cucumbers, diced

1/4 cup red onion, chopped

1/4 cup feta cheese crumbles

2/TBS of olive oil

1-tablespoon lemon juice

pepper and salt as desired

Instructions

• Combine the cooked quinoa, mixed greens, cherry tomatoes, diced cucumber, and diced red onion in a sizable mixing dish.

• Combine the olive oil and lemon juice thoroughly in a separate small bowl.

• Add the dressing to the bowl and stir to combine.

Feta cheese crumbles are added to the bowl, and salt and pepper are added to taste.

Grilled Portobello Mushroom Burger

Ingredients

2 substantial portobellos

1 tablespoon of olive oil

pepper and salt as desired

two whole-wheat buns

14 cup of red onion slices

14 cup of chopped avocado

1/9 cup mustard

Instructions

• Heat a grill or grill pan to a moderately high temperature.

Olive oil should be brushed on the portobello mushrooms, and salt and pepper should be added.

• Grill the mushrooms for 5 to 7 minutes on each side, or until they are soft and gently browned.

• Grill the buns for a brief period of time.

On the bottom half of each bread, spread mustard.

• Place a grilled mushroom and a slice of red onion or avocado on each bread.

• Place the second half of the bun on top, then serve.

Tacos With Black Beans And Sweet Potatoes

Ingredients

two medium sweet potatoes, diced after being peeled

1 tablespoon of olive oil

1 teaspoon cumin, ground

Chili powder, 1/2 tsp.

pepper and salt as desired

1 can of rinsed and drained black beans

1/4 cup red onion, chopped

14 cup finely minced fresh cilantro

1 lime's juice

6 tortillas de maiz

Instructions

Set the oven's temperature to 400 °F.

Spread out on a baking sheet, toss the diced sweet potatoes with the olive oil, cumin, chili powder, salt, and pepper, and roast for 20 to 25 minutes, or until soft and just beginning to caramelize.

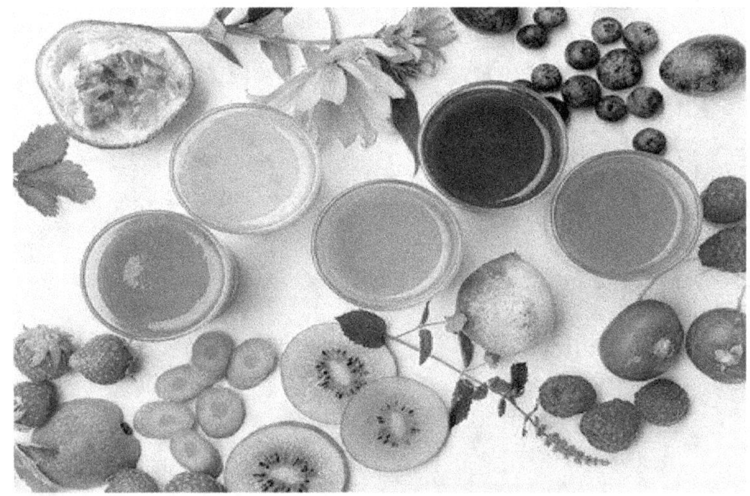

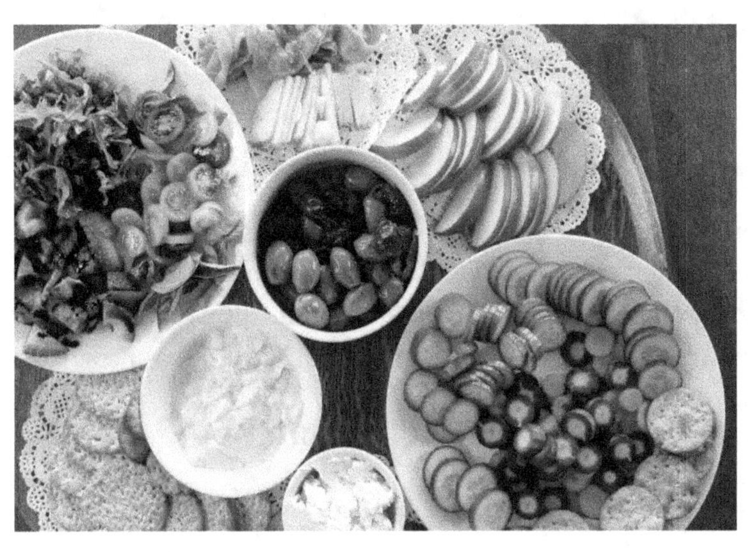

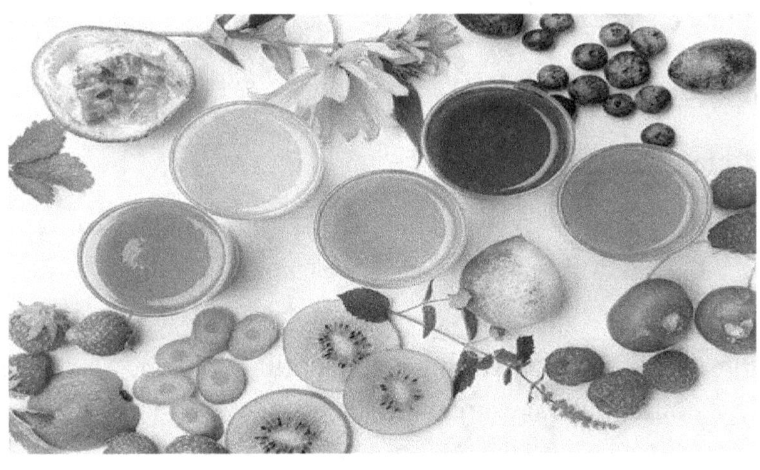

CHAPTER 5

SALADS AND DRESSINGS

Alkaline foods can be added to salads to balance your diet. They are simple to prepare, adaptable, and may be customized to your tastes. Here are some recipes for and dressing ideas for alkaline salads:

Strawberry And Spinach Salad

Ingredients

4 cups of young spinach

1 cup of strawberry slices

14 cup of almond slices

1/4 cup feta cheese crumbles

Balsamic vinegar, 2 tbsp.

1 tablespoon of honey

2/TBS of olive oil

Instructions

Baby spinach, sliced strawberries, sliced almonds, and feta cheese crumbles should all be combined in a big bowl.

Whisk the balsamic vinegar, honey, and olive oil together in a separate small basin.

Toss the salad with the dressing after pouring it over it.

Cucumber And Tomato Salad

Ingredients

2 sliced cucumbers, 1 pint of cherry tomatoes, and

1/4 cup red onion, chopped

2 tbsp freshly chopped parsley

2/TBS of olive oil

1-tablespoon lemon juice

pepper and salt as desired

Instructions

• Combine the diced red onion, cherry tomatoes, cucumber slices, and parsley in a sizable mixing dish.

• Combine the olive oil and lemon juice thoroughly in a separate small bowl.

• Drizzle the salad with the dressing and toss to combine.

Add salt and pepper to taste when seasoning.

Salad Of Kale And Quinoa

Ingredients

4 cups of kale, chopped

cooked quinoa, 1 cup

chopped walnuts, half a cup

14 cup of dried cranberries

Apple cider vinegar, 2 tablespoons

1 tablespoon of honey

2/TBS of olive oil

Instructions

Combine the cooked quinoa, chopped walnuts, dried cranberries, and chopped kale in a large bowl.

• Mix the apple cider vinegar, honey, and olive oil together in a separate small basin.

• Drizzle the salad with the dressing and toss to combine.

Avocado And Tomato Salad

Ingredients

2 diced avocados

1 pint of halved cherry tomatoes

1/4 cup red onion, chopped

2 tbsp freshly chopped cilantro

1.5 tbsp lime juice

2/TBS of olive oil

pepper and salt as desired

Instructions

• Combine the diced avocados, cherry tomatoes, red onion, and cilantro in a sizable mixing dish.

• Combine the lime juice and olive oil thoroughly in a separate small bowl.

• Drizzle the salad with the dressing and toss to combine.

Add salt and pepper to taste when seasoning.

Lemon And Garlic Dressing

Ingredients

1/8 cup lemon juice, fresh

Olive oil, 1/4 cup

2 minced garlic cloves

pepper and salt as desired

Instructions

• Combine the lemon juice, olive oil, and minced garlic in a small bowl. Whisk until thoroughly blended.

Add salt and pepper to taste when seasoning.

Balsamic Vinaigrette Dressing

Ingredients

Balsamic vinegar, 1/4 cup

Olive oil, 1/4 cup

Dijon mustard, 1 teaspoon

1 minced garlic clove

pepper and salt as desired

Instructions

• Combine the balsamic vinegar, olive oil, Dijon mustard, and minced garlic in a small bowl. Whisk until thoroughly blended.

• Add salt and pepper to taste when seasoning.

The pH Scale

Gastric acid
Lemon juice
Apple juice
Tomato juice
Black coffee
Milk
Pure water
Egg
Baking soda
Hand soap
Ammonia solution
BLEACH
Bleach
Concentrated solutions of alkalis
1 2 3 4 5 6 7 8 9 10 11 12 13 14
ACID
NEUTRAL
BASE

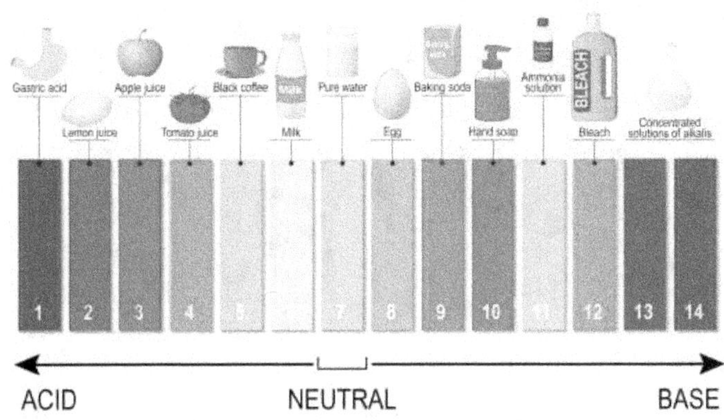

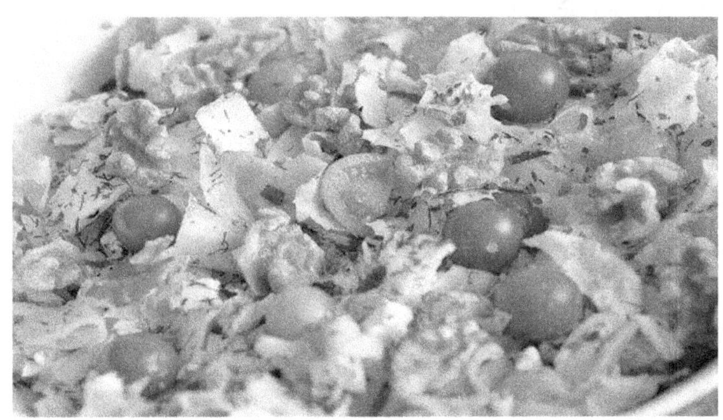

CHAPTER 6

SOUPS AND STEWS

A healthy and soothing approach to include alkaline foods in your diet is through soups and stews. Here are some recipes for alkaline soup and stew to try:

Vegetable Soup

Ingredients

1 can of diced tomatoes and 4 cups of vegetable broth

2 cups of chopped veggies, such as zucchini, carrots, and celery

cooked quinoa, 1 cup

Dry thyme, 1 teaspoon

Dried oregano, 1 teaspoon

pepper and salt as desired

Instructions

• Bring the vegetable broth to a simmer in a big pot.

Add the cooked quinoa, dried thyme, and dried oregano, along with the diced tomatoes, chopped veggies, and salt and pepper to taste.

• Simmer the vegetables for 20 to 30 minutes, or until they are soft.

Lentil Stew

Ingredients

two cups of vegetable stock

1 cup dried lentils, drained after rinsing

1 tomato diced can

1 diced onion, 3 minced garlic cloves

2 cups of finely chopped vegetables, such as sweet potatoes, carrots, and celery

Dry thyme, 1 teaspoon

pepper and salt as desired

Instructions

• Bring the vegetable broth to a simmer in a big pot.

• Include the lentils, chopped veggies, diced tomatoes, onion, garlic, and dry thyme.

Add salt and pepper to taste when seasoning.

• Simmer the lentils and vegetables for 30 to 40 minutes, or until they are soft.

Butternut Squash Soup

Ingredients

1 medium butternut squash, diced after being peeled

1 diced onion, 2 minced garlic cloves

4 cups of veggie broth

Dry thyme, 1 teaspoon

50 ml of coconut milk

pepper and salt as desired

Instructions

• Saute the butternut squash, onion, and garlic in a big pot until the vegetables are soft.

• Include the dried thyme and veggie broth.

• Simmer the butternut squash for 20 to 30 minutes, or until it is tender.

• Puree the soup using an immersion blender until it is smooth.

Add the coconut milk and season to taste with salt and pepper.

White Bean and Kale Soup

Ingredients

4 cups of veggie broth

1 can of washed and drained white beans

2 cups of kale, chopped

1 diced onion, 3 minced garlic cloves

Dried oregano, 1 teaspoon

0.5 teaspoon of red pepper flakes

pepper and salt as desired

Instructions

Sauté the onion and garlic in a large pot until the vegetables are soft.

• Include the white beans, chopped kale, dry oregano, and red pepper flakes along with the vegetable broth.

• Let the kale simmer for 20 to 30 minutes, or until it wilts.

Add salt and pepper to taste when seasoning.

Tomato and Basil Soup

Ingredients

4 cups of veggie broth

1 tomato diced can

1 diced onion, 3 minced garlic cloves

Chopped fresh basil, half a cup

50 ml of coconut milk

pepper and salt as desired

Instructions

• with a big pot, cook the vegetables with the onion and garlic until they are soft.

• Include the veggie broth along with the diced tomatoes and basil.

• Simmer the tomatoes for 20 to 30 minutes, or until they are tender.

• Puree the soup using an immersion blender until it is smooth.

Add the coconut milk and season to taste with salt and pepper.

Minestrone Soup

Ingredients

4 cups of veggie broth

1 tomato diced can

1 diced onion, 3 minced garlic cloves

2 cups of chopped veggies, such as zucchini, carrots, and celery

1 can of washed and drained white beans

Dried oregano, 1 teaspoon

pepper and salt as desired

Instructions

• with a big pot, cook the vegetables with the onion and garlic until they are soft.

White beans, diced tomatoes, chopped veggies, vegetable broth, dry oregano, and white beans should all be added.

• Simmer the vegetables for 20 to 30 minutes, or until they are tender.

Add salt and pepper to taste when seasoning.

Chickpea And Spinach Stew

Ingredients

4 cups of veggie broth

1 can of washed and drained chickpeas

2 cups of spinach, chopped

1 diced onion, 3 minced garlic cloves

Smoked paprika, 1 teaspoon

12 teaspoon cumin

pepper and salt as desired

Instructions

• with a big pot, cook the vegetables with the onion and garlic until they are soft.

• Include the chickpeas, chopped spinach, cumin, smoked paprika, and vegetable broth.

• Simmer for 20 to 30 minutes, or until the spinach wilts and the chickpeas are tender.

Add salt and pepper to taste when seasoning.

Carrot And Ginger Soup

Ingredients

4 cups of veggie broth

4 cups of carrots, chopped

3 cloves of minced garlic, 1 inch piece of peeled and grated fresh ginger, 1 onion, chopped

50 ml of coconut milk

pepper and salt as desired

Instructions

Sauté the onion, garlic, and ginger in a large pot until the vegetables are soft.

• Include the chopped carrots and the vegetable broth.

• Simmer the carrots for 20 to 30 minutes, or until they are tender.

• Puree the soup using an immersion blender until it is smooth.

Add the coconut milk and season to taste with salt and pepper.

Miso Soup

Ingredients

4 cups vegetarian broth 1 diced block of firm tofu

Chopped green onions, half a cup

Miso paste, 1/4 cup

1 teaspoon sesame oil

pepper and salt as desired

Instructions

• Bring the vegetable broth to a simmer in a big pot.

• Include the chopped green onions and tofu cubes.

• Miso paste and a little hot water should be combined in a small bowl and whisked until smooth.

Stir the miso mixture into the soup after adding it.

• Simmer for 5 to 10 minutes, or until thoroughly cooked.

Add the sesame oil and season to taste with salt and pepper.

Beet and Potato Soup

Ingredients

4 cups vegetable broth

2 cups chopped beets

2 cups chopped potatoes

1 onion, chopped

3 cloves garlic, minced

1 tsp dried thyme

Salt and pepper to taste

Instructions

- In a large pot, sauté the onion and garlic until the vegetables are tender.

- Add the vegetable broth, chopped beets, chopped potatoes, and dried thyme.

- Simmer for 20-30 minutes or until the vegetables are soft.

- Use an immersion blender to puree the soup until smooth.

- Wraps and sandwiches

Grilled Vegetable Wrap

Ingredients

1 large tortilla wrap

1/2 zucchini, sliced

1/2 red bell pepper, sliced

1/2 yellow bell pepper, sliced

1/2 red onion, sliced

1 tbsp olive oil

Salt and pepper to taste

2 tbsp hummus

Handful of mixed greens

Instructions

- Preheat a grill pan or skillet over medium-high heat.

- Toss the sliced vegetables in olive oil and season with salt and pepper.

- Grill the vegetables for 3-4 minutes on each side until they are slightly charred and tender.

- Spread the hummus onto the tortilla wrap.

- Add the mixed greens and grilled vegetables.

- Roll up the wrap tightly and cut in half before serving.

Avocado and Tofu Sandwich

Ingredients

2 slices of bread (gluten-free or whole grain)

1/2 avocado, mashed

4 oz firm tofu, sliced

1 tbsp olive oil

1 tsp smoked paprika

Salt and pepper to taste

Handful of arugula

Instructions

- Heat the olive oil in a skillet over medium-high heat.

- Add the sliced tofu and sprinkle with smoked paprika, salt, and pepper.

- Cook for 3-4 minutes on each side until the tofu is crispy and golden brown.

- Toast the bread slices.

- Spread the mashed avocado onto one slice of bread.

- Add the arugula and cooked tofu.

- Top with the other slice of bread and cut in half before serving.

Greek Wrap

Ingredients

1 large tortilla wrap

4 oz grilled chicken or tofu, sliced

1/4 cup diced cucumber

1/4 cup diced tomato

1/4 cup crumbled feta cheese

2 tbsp tzatziki sauce

Handful of mixed greens

Instructions

- Lay the tortilla wrap flat on a plate.

- Spread the tzatziki sauce onto the tortilla wrap.

- Add the mixed greens, sliced chicken or tofu, diced cucumber, diced tomato, and crumbled feta cheese.

- Roll up the wrap tightly and cut in half before serving.

Quinoa and Veggie Wrap

Ingredients

1 large tortilla wrap

1/2 cup cooked quinoa

1/2 cup chopped veggies (such as bell peppers, carrots, and zucchini)

2 tbsp hummus

Handful of mixed greens

Salt and pepper to taste

Instructions

Lay the tortilla wrap flat on a plate.

Spread the hummus onto the tortilla wrap.

Add the cooked quinoa, mixed greens, and chopped veggies.

Season with salt and pepper to taste.

Roll up the wrap tightly and cut in half before serving.

Caprese Sandwich

Ingredients

2 slices of bread (gluten-free or whole grain)

1/2 cup sliced tomato

1/4 cup sliced fresh mozzarella cheese

Handful of fresh basil leaves

1 tbsp balsamic vinegar

Salt and pepper to taste

Instructions

- Toast the bread slices.

- Layer the sliced tomato, fresh mozzarella cheese, and fresh basil leaves onto one slice of bread.

- Drizzle with balsamic vinegar and season with salt and pepper to taste.

- Top with the other slice of bread and cut in half before serving.

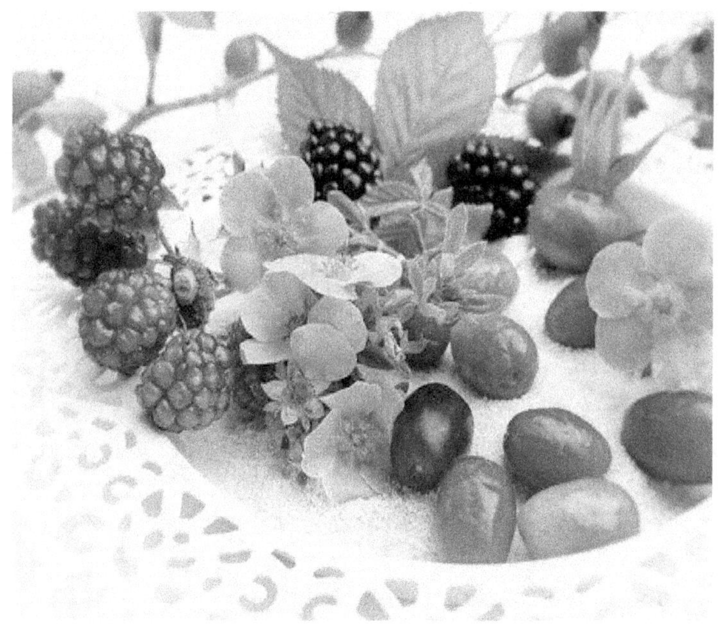

CHAPTER 7

RECIPES FOR ALKALINE DINNERS

The goal of an acid-alkaline diet is to balance your body's pH level by eating foods that have an alkaline effect. Vegetables, fruits, whole grains, nuts, and seeds are some of the low-acid, high-alkaline items that make up the diet.

Here are some alkaline dinner recipes that are not only scrumptious but also healthful.

Salmon is marinated in a mixture of lemon juice, olive oil, garlic, and herbs before being baked. Serve with roasted veggies after baking in the oven until thoroughly done.

Quinoa stir-fry: Prepare the quinoa as directed on the package, then stir-fry it with a range of vibrant veggies like peppers, carrots, and zucchini.

Vegetable skewers that have been grilled: Thread a variety of vibrant veggies, like cherry tomatoes, mushrooms, and bell peppers, onto skewers and cook over a hot grill until they are soft.

Cook onions, garlic, and ginger in olive oil for a vegan chickpea curry. Include diced tomatoes, chickpeas, and a curry spice mixture. Over brown rice, please.

Sweet potatoes should be cut into wedges and tossed with salt, pepper, and olive oil for baked sweet potato fries. Bake till crispy in the oven.

Until the cauliflower florets resemble rice, process them in a food processor to make stir-fried cauliflower rice. Various colored veggies are sautéed with garlic, onion, and other seasonings.

Sauté onions, garlic, and ginger in olive oil before making vegan lentil soup. Add a mixture of spices along with the lentils, diced tomatoes, and vegetable broth. Till the lentils are cooked, simmer.

Marinate portobello mushrooms in a mixture of balsamic vinegar, olive oil, garlic, and herbs before grilling. Serve with a side salad after being grilled till soft.

Sauté peppers, onions, and garlic in olive oil for a vegan quinoa chili. Mix in some quinoa, chopped tomatoes, vegetable broth, and a mixture of chili seasonings. Till the quinoa is cooked, simmer.

Vegetable kebabs with grilled tofu can be made by skewering tofu, bell peppers, onions, and zucchini.

Remove the tops and seeds from bell peppers before stuffing them with vegan ingredients. Place quinoa, black beans, diced tomatoes, and seasonings inside. Until soft, bake in the oven.

Olive oil-based vegan butternut squash soup with sautéed onions, garlic, and ginger. Add a mixture of spices, butternut squash, and vegetable broth. Simmer the squash until it's soft. until smooth, puree.

Pizza with grilled vegetables: Add grilled peppers, zucchini, and eggplant to a whole-wheat pizza crust. The crust should be baked in the oven until crisp.

Make a vegan shepherd's pie with lentils by sautéing onions, garlic, and carrots in oil. Add a mixture of herbs, cooked lentils, and vegetable broth. Add mashed sweet potatoes on top, then bake until bubbling.

Vegetarian lasagna with roasted veggies: Layer lasagna noodles, vegan cheese, and roasted vegetables including eggplant, zucchini, and bell peppers. Bake till bubbling in the oven.

Chili made using vegan black beans and sweet potatoes: Sauté peppers, onions, and garlic in olive oil. Diced sweet potatoes, diced tomatoes, and a mixture of chili spices should all be added. Until the sweet potatoes are cooked through, simmer.

Vegetables like broccoli, tomatoes, and peppers can be roasted for a vegan quiche. In a pie crust, combine with a vegan egg substitute, and bake until firm.

Wraps made with grilled veggies: Grilled vegetables include onions, zucchini, and eggplant. Using whole-grain tortillas, hummus, avocado, and fresh herbs, wrap them.

Cut a head of cauliflower into thick slices and brush with a mixture of olive oil, garlic, and herbs for a vegan roasted cauliflower steak. Until soft, roast in the oven and serve with a side salad.

Sauté onions, garlic, and ginger in olive oil for a vegan stew with spinach and chickpeas. Diced tomatoes, spinach, chickpeas, and a mixture of spices should be added. Simmer until the chickpeas are thoroughly warm and the spinach has wilted.

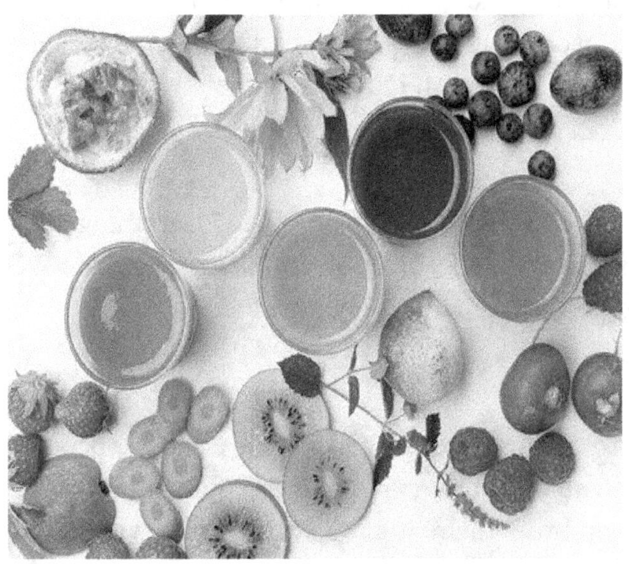

CHAPTER 8

OTHER ALKALINE RECIPES

VEGETABLE-BASED MAINS

Making delicious and healthy meals with a vegetable base is a terrific approach to increase your intake of veggies. Here are ten vegetable-based main dish ideas that are sure to impress.

Bowls of roasted vegetables and quinoa: Roast a range of vegetables, including sweet potatoes, broccoli, and Brussels sprouts. Serve with quinoa and pour some tahini sauce on top.

Black beans, quinoa, and roasted veggies like peppers, onions, and zucchini can all be combined to make veggie burgers. Make patties, then bake or broil them until crispy. Serve with your preferred toppings on a whole-grain bun.

Sauté tomatoes, eggplant, zucchini, and other vegetables with onions, garlic, and other seasonings to make ratatouille. Serve with quinoa or brown rice.

Remove the stems from portobello mushrooms and load the interior with a mixture of quinoa that has been cooked, sliced tomatoes, and spinach. Until soft, bake in the oven.

Sauté bell peppers, green beans, onions, garlic, and other veggies for the vegetarian paella. Short-grain rice should be cooked until it is soft before adding saffron. Lemon wedges are recommended.

Stir-fry with zucchini noodles: Spiralize zucchini to make noodles, then toss them in a pan with garlic, onions, and a range of vibrant veggies including carrots and bell peppers. Serve with a splash of teriyaki or soy sauce.

Olive oil is used to sauté onions, garlic, and carrots for lentil shepherd's pie. Add a mixture of herbs, cooked lentils, and vegetable broth. Add mashed sweet potatoes on top, then bake until bubbling.

Sauté onions, garlic, and ginger in olive oil for the sweet potato curry. Add coconut milk, sliced sweet potatoes, and a mixture of curry spices. Until the sweet potatoes are cooked through, simmer. Over brown rice, please.

Vegetarian enchiladas: Stuff corn tortillas with a mixture of roasted bell peppers, onions, chopped tomatoes, and black beans. Enchilada sauce should be added, then bake until bubbling.

Vegetable lasagna: Combine lasagna noodles, cheese, or a vegan cheese substitute, with roasted veggies including eggplant, zucchini, and bell peppers. Bake till bubbling in the oven.

These major dishes made of vegetables are flavorful, nutrient-dense, and guaranteed to sate your hunger. Try incorporating these dishes into your meal plan for a healthier you. Adding more veggies to your diet will help you maintain a healthy weight and lower your chance of developing chronic diseases.

SEAFOOD AND FISH DISHES

Fish and seafood are healthful additions to any diet because they are excellent providers of lean protein and omega-3 fatty acids. These fish and seafood meals can be made in accordance with an acid-alkaline diet.

Salmon fillets are seasoned with lemon juice, olive oil, and fresh dill when they are grilled. Serve hot off the grill with roasted vegetables on the side.

Cod fillets are seasoned with garlic, tomatoes, and olives in a baked dish. Serve the fish with a dish of quinoa or brown rice after baking it in the oven until it is fully cooked.

Shrimp sautéed in olive oil with garlic and lemon juice is known as lemon-garlic shrimp. Serve over quinoa or brown rice and a bed of mixed greens.

Scallops with spinach that have been pan-seared in olive oil and served with a squeeze of lemon juice.

Avocado-tuna salad: Combine canned tuna, mashed avocado, lemon juice, and celery. Serve with tomatoes and cucumbers on a bed of mixed greens.

Swordfish steaks are seasoned with a mixture of spices and grilled until fully done, served with mango salsa. Serve alongside a dish of cilantro, red onion, and sliced mango salsa.

Cod fillets are seasoned with lemon juice, olive oil, and a combination of fresh herbs before being baked. Serve the fish with a side of roasted veggies after baking in the oven until the fish is thoroughly done.

Sea salt the salmon fillets before broiling them. Serve the salmon with steamed asparagus and a side of quinoa or brown rice.

Shrimp with a Variety of Colorful Vegetables Stir-Fried: Stir-fry shrimp with bell peppers, onions, and a variety of colorful vegetables, such as broccoli. Serve over a bed of brown rice or quinoa.

Sliced cucumbers, radishes, and sesame oil are added to a side salad that is served with seared tuna steaks that have been cooked in olive oil.

These seafood and fish recipes are not only mouthwatering, but they also help you keep a healthy acid-alkaline balance in your diet. You may benefit from the health advantages of fish and seafood while keeping your body alkaline by including these recipes in your diet plan.

MEAT AND POULTRY DISHES

As long as they are consumed in moderation and prepared healthily, meat and poultry can also be included in an acid-alkaline diet. These recipes for meat and poultry dishes are appropriate for an acid-alkaline diet.

Chicken breasts should be marinated in lemon juice, olive oil, and fresh thyme before being baked. Serve with a side of roasted veggies after baking in the oven until thoroughly heated through.

Chicken breasts are seasoned with a blend of spices and grilled until fully cooked. This dish is served with mango salsa. Serve alongside a dish of cilantro, red onion, and sliced mango salsa.

To make turkey meatballs with tomato sauce, combine the chopped herbs, onions, and garlic with the ground turkey. Make meatballs out of the mixture, then bake them in the oven until done. Serve alongside a dish of homemade tomato sauce made from chopped tomatoes and fresh herbs.

Beef and Veggie Stir-Fry: Stir-fry a range of colorful veggies, including bell peppers, onions, and broccoli with strips of beef. Serve over a bed of brown rice or quinoa.

Salmon fillets and chicken breasts can be marinated in a mixture of lemon juice, olive oil, and fresh herbs before being baked. Serve with a side of roasted veggies after baking in the oven until thoroughly heated through.

Ground turkey, sliced avocado, and a mixture of seasonings are combined to make grilled turkey burgers. Make patties, then grill them until done. Serve with your preferred toppings on a whole-grain bun.

Ground turkey, onions, garlic, and olive oil are sautéed in a chili recipe. Beans, tomatoes, and a mixture of chili spices should be added. Simmer the chili until it is steaming and bubbling.

Beef and Broccoli Stir-Fry: Combine beef strips, broccoli, and a variety of seasonings in a stir-fry. Serve over a bed of brown rice or quinoa.

Chicken and Vegetable Skewers: Thread cherry tomatoes, zucchini, and other vibrant veggies, along with chicken breast, onto skewers. Serve with quinoa or brown rice as a side dish after grilling until thoroughly cooked.

Baked Turkey and Vegetable Casserole: In a casserole dish, arrange slices of sweet potatoes, bell peppers, zucchini, and other vibrant veggies. Serve with quinoa or brown rice as a side dish and bake in the oven until thoroughly done.

These protein- and flavor-rich poultry and beef recipes are great for preserving the acid-alkaline balance in your diet. You may keep your body in an alkaline condition while receiving the health advantages of lean protein by integrating these recipes into your diet routine.

SIDE DISHES AND SNACKS

Any diet must include snacks and side dishes, and there are many choices that are appropriate for an acid-alkaline diet. Here are some recipes for appetizers and sides that will keep your body's pH level alkaline.

Cauliflower Roasted: Toss cauliflower florets with sea salt and olive oil. Roast till crisp and golden brown in the oven.

Slice the zucchini into thin rounds, then mix with sea salt and olive oil to make zucchini chips. Serve as a nutritious substitute for potato chips after baking in the oven until crispy.

Blend roasted beets with chickpeas, tahini, lemon juice, and garlic to make roasted beet hummus. Serve with whole-grain crackers or sliced vegetables.

Brussels sprouts that have been roasted are tossed in olive oil and sea salt. Bake something till it becomes crispy and caramelized.

Kale Chips: Toss chopped kale with sea salt and olive oil. Serve as a nutritious substitute for potato chips after baking in the oven until crispy.

Quinoa salad: Prepare the quinoa per the instructions on the package, then combine with chopped vegetables like cucumber, bell pepper, and cherry tomatoes. Lemon juice and olive oil are used to dress.

Sweet potato wedges should be tossed with olive oil and sea salt for roasting. As a nutritious substitute for French fries, roast until crispy in the oven.

Blend roasted eggplant with tahini, lemon juice, garlic, and olive oil to make baba ghanoush. Serve with whole-grain crackers or sliced vegetables.

Broccoli that has been steam-cooked should be bright green and soft. Add a dash of olive oil and sea salt before serving.

Sliced cucumber should be combined with diced red onion, cherry tomatoes, and sea salt in a cucumber salad. Lemon juice and olive oil are used to dress.

These appetizers and sides are not only tasty, but they also help you keep a healthy acid-alkaline balance in your diet. You can have wholesome and filling snacks and side dishes while keeping your body in an alkaline state by including these recipes in your meal plan.

SODIUM-FREE SNACKS & DIPS

Here are some alkaline-friendly recipes for dips and snacks that are ideal for an acid-alkaline diet.

Serve a dish of sliced raw veggies including carrots, celery, bell peppers, and cucumbers along with a side of homemade hummus that is made with chickpeas, tahini, and lemon juice.

Ripe avocados are blended with sliced tomatoes, red onion, cilantro, and carrot sticks to make guacamole. For a balanced and healthful snack, serve alongside carrot sticks.

Sweet potatoes are sliced into small circles and baked in the oven until crispy. They are served with a cashew dip. Serve with a dip of cashews, lemon juice, and herbs that have been soaked.

Slice the zucchini into thin ribbons with a vegetable peeler to make raw zucchini rolls. On each ribbon, apply a small layer of cashew cheese before rolling.

Use a vegetable peeler to slice the cucumber into thin strips for the cucumber and avocado sushi rolls. Place the cucumber strips on a nori sheet, then add the mashed avocado on top. Slice into bite-sized pieces after rolling.

Apple Slices with Raw Almond Butter: For a filling and alkaline snack, spread apple slices with raw almond butter.

Lay a sheet of nori on a flat surface. Spread a thin layer of hummus or cashew cheese over the nori. Sliced raw veggies like bell peppers, carrots, and cucumbers can be added on top. Slice into bite-sized pieces after rolling.

White bean and roasted beet dip: This vibrant and nutritious dip is made by blending white beans, roasted beets, lemon juice, and herbs.

Raw Almond and Date Balls: Combine dates, raw almonds, and a dash of sea salt. Make bite-sized balls out of the mixture and eat as a sweet and filling alkaline snack.

Toss kale leaves in olive oil and sea salt before serving with spicy salsa as raw kale chips. Serve with a side of hot salsa made with diced tomatoes, onions, and herbs after baking till crispy in the oven.

In addition to being nutritious and delectable, these alkaline snacks and dips are excellent for preserving your body's alkaline balance. You can have a variety of gratifying and alkaline snacks and dips that will make you feel your best if you include these recipes in your meal plan.

For a flavorful and alkaline soup, combine raw carrots, ginger, apple cider vinegar, and spices.

Raw broccoli and walnut dip: For a tasty and alkaline dip, blend raw broccoli florets with walnuts, olive oil, lemon juice, and herbs.

Chickpeas should be mixed with spices, olive oil, and oil. Enjoy as a nutritious and alkaline snack after roasting in the oven until crispy.

A rich and flavorful pâté can be made by blending raw mushrooms, walnuts, olive oil, lemon juice, and seasonings.

Kale and White Bean Dip: To make this creamy, alkaline dip, combine cooked white beans, cooked kale, garlic, olive oil, and lemon juice.

Raw Red Pepper and Almond Dip: For a sweet and tangy dip, combine raw red peppers with almonds, olive oil, lemon juice, and spices.

Raw Cucumber and Dill Dip: For a reviving and alkaline dip, blend raw cucumbers with fresh dill, cashews, lemon juice, and spices.

Raw Beet and Carrot Salad: For a vibrant and alkaline salad, shred raw beets and carrots and combine with a dressing of olive oil, lemon juice, and spices.

Raw Spinach and Avocado Dip: For a creamy, alkaline dip, blend raw spinach, ripe avocados, lemon juice, garlic, and spices.

Slice eggplant into thin rounds and bake until crispy with basil dip for baked eggplant chips. For a delectable and alkaline snack, serve with a dip made with fresh basil, garlic, olive oil, and lemon juice.

You'll have even more variety and alternatives for filling and healthful snacks that support an alkaline balance in your body if you include these extra alkaline snacks and dips in your meal plan.

FOR MEALS, SIDE DISHES

Asparagus is roasted with lemon and tossed in olive oil before being baked till soft. Just before serving, squeeze some fresh lemon juice on top.

Quinoa Pilaf with Vegetables: Saute onions, bell peppers, and zucchini with the quinoa while it cooks in vegetable broth.

Swiss chard with Garlic Sautéd: For a quick and tasty side meal, sauté Swiss chard in olive oil with garlic and lemon juice.

Brussels sprouts are roasted in the oven with balsamic vinegar after being coated in olive oil. Before serving, drizzle with balsamic vinegar.

Garlic, lemon juice, and olive oil are added to steamed broccoli after it has been cooked till tender.

Cauliflower is roasted with turmeric and tossed in olive oil before being baked till crispy.

Root veggies can be roasted by tossing a variety of them in olive oil and roasting them in the oven until they are fork-tender.

Apple cider vinegar, Dijon mustard, and maple syrup are combined to make a homemade apple cider vinaigrette, which is then drizzled over kale after it has been massaged with olive oil.

Grilled eggplant with herbs: Brush slices of eggplant with oil, then grill until they are soft. Add fresh herbs like parsley and basil on top.

Cinnamon-Rubbed Baked Sweet Potato Wedges: Cut sweet potatoes into wedges and bake them in the oven until they are crisp. Before serving, add a cinnamon sprinkling.

SUITABLE DESSERTS

Apples should be cored and baked with cinnamon until they are soft. Add some cinnamon, then indulge!

Chia Seed Pudding: Combine the chia seeds with the almond milk, honey, and vanilla essence. Enjoy it as a nutritious and alkaline pudding after letting it settle in the refrigerator over night.

A rich and indulgent dessert, raw chocolate avocado mousse is made by blending ripe avocados with raw cacao powder, honey, and vanilla extract.

Fresh Berries with Coconut Cream: For a delectable and alkaline dessert, top fresh berries with whipped coconut cream and a dusting of coconut sugar.

Peaches should be cut in half and roasted in the oven until soft. Serve with yogurt. Serve with a drizzle of honey and plain yogurt.

The base and filling for a raw and alkaline cheesecake are made from a mixture of cashews, dates, and blueberries.

Almond milk, vanilla extract, and frozen bananas are blended to create a creamy, alkaline ice cream.

Halve the pears and sprinkle with almond meal, cinnamon, and honey for baked pears with almonds. Enjoy as a wholesome and alkaline dessert after baking in the oven until soft.

Lemon Bars with Almond Flour Crust: To prepare the crust, combine almond flour, coconut oil, and honey. Add a lemon filling on top that was produced with eggs, lemon juice, and honey.

Blend shredded coconut, coconut oil, honey, and vanilla extract to make raw coconut macaroons. Form into balls and chill until solid.

Make raw almond butter cups by combining raw cacao powder, coconut oil, and honey with almond butter. Fill muffin tins with the mixture, then freeze until solid.

Pears should be poached in water with cinnamon and honey. Serve with vanilla yogurt. Add some vanilla essence and plain yogurt to the dish before serving.

Almonds, dates, and coconut oil are combined to produce the crust for a raw raspberry tart. Add a cashew, raspberry, and honey filling as the garnish.

Sliced pineapple is grilled with coconut cream until it is soft. Add some coconut sugar and whipped coconut cream over top.

Chia seeds should be combined with almond milk, raw cacao powder, and honey to make chocolate chia seed pudding. Enjoy it as a healthy, alkaline chocolate pudding after letting it lie in the refrigerator over night.

Cashews, dates, and strawberries are blended to create the base and filling of a raw, alkaline cheesecake.

Apples stuffed with cinnamon and topped with oat crumble are baked. The crumble is made of oats, coconut oil, and honey. Until soft, bake in the oven.

Blend frozen mango with coconut milk, honey, and lime juice to make coconut mango sorbet. Enjoy as an alkaline and nutritious sorbet after freezing until solid.

Almond flour, eggs, coconut oil, honey, and blueberries are combined to make lemon blueberry muffins. Enjoy an alkaline and nutritious muffin after baking till fluffy.

Raw carrot cake bites: To make the base, blend the carrots, dates, coconut, and spices. Form into balls and chill until solid. To create an alkaline and nutritious carrot cake bite, top with cashew cream icing.

These treats are a delightful way to sate your sweet desire while keeping your body's pH levels alkaline. You can enjoy a range of healthy and alkaline sweets if you include these recipes in your food plan.

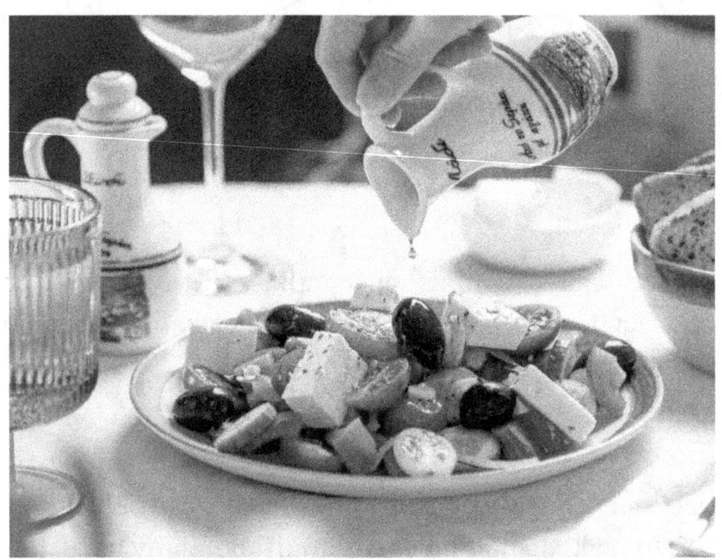

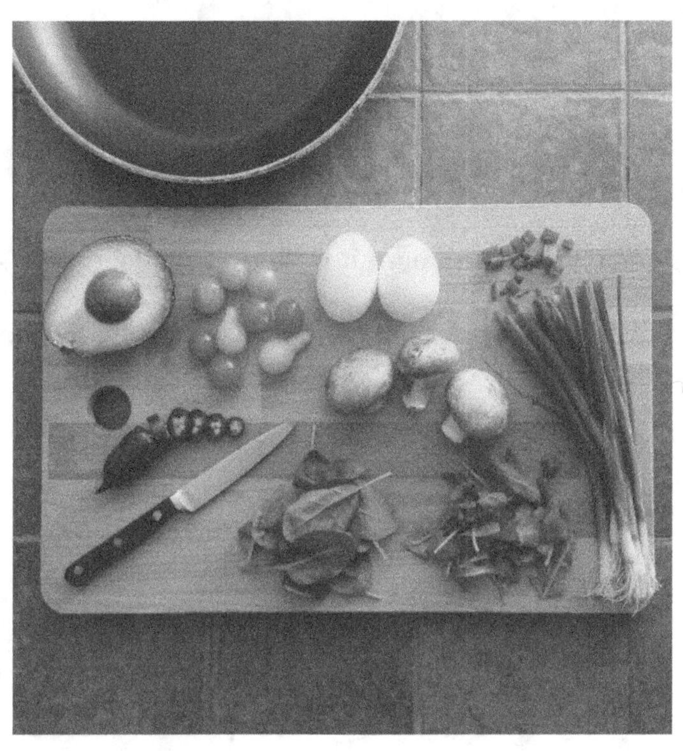

CHAPTER 9

SPECIAL OCCASION RECIPES

Cook the salmon on the grill until it is thoroughly done, then serve it with an avocado salsa prepared of chopped avocado, tomato, red onion, lime juice, and cilantro.

Quinoa-stuffed portobello mushrooms are stuffed with a mixture of quinoa, spinach, garlic, and feta cheese after being roasted.

Roasted Turkey with Rosemary and Lemon: For a tasty and alkaline main dish, roast turkey with rosemary and lemon.

Alkaline Caesar Salad: Combine romaine lettuce, olive oil, lemon juice, garlic, and anchovy paste in an alkaline Caesar dressing. Add some Parmesan cheese and croutons made from bread that has been sprouted.

Cashews, coconut oil, dates, and vanilla extract are combined to create the base and filling of a raw, vegan cheesecake. For a dessert fit for a special occasion, top with fresh berries.

Cooking brown rice in a vegetable broth flavored with saffron and adding sautéed vegetables such bell peppers, onions, and artichoke hearts results in an alkaline vegetable paella. Lemon wedges and fresh parsley go on top.

Lamb chops are grilled until they are cooked to your preference, then they are topped with a mint pesto that is made with fresh mint, garlic, lemon juice, and olive oil.

Raw Vegan Chocolate Truffles: To make a decadent and rich chocolate truffle, combine soaked cashews, dates, cocoa powder, and coconut oil. For an added touch, roll in chopped nuts or shredded coconut.

Alkaline Ratatouille: Arrange tomato, eggplant, and zucchini slices in a baking dish together with herbs and olive oil. Roast till flavorful and tender.

Smooth and creamy alkaline chocolate mousse can be made by blending avocado, unprocessed cacao powder, maple syrup, and vanilla extract. For a delicious dessert, top with fresh berries.

When you want to wow your guests or prepare a special supper for your loved ones, these recipes are ideal. You may prepare meals that are tasty, healthful, and beneficial to your body by employing alkaline ingredients and techniques.

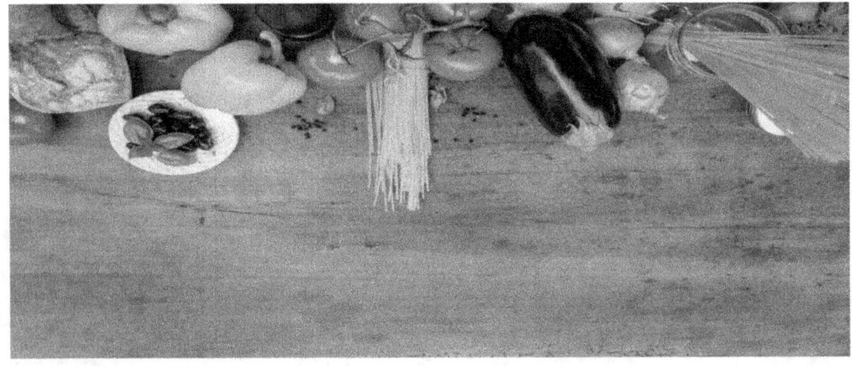

RECIPES FOR ALKALINE HOLIDAYS

Alkaline Roasted Turkey: For a tasty and alkaline main dish, roast a turkey with rosemary and lemon.

Alkaline Cranberry Sauce: For a sweet and tangy side dish, cook fresh cranberries with orange juice, cinnamon, and stevia.

Sweet potatoes should be boiled until they are tender before being mashed with almond milk, cinnamon, and a tiny bit of maple syrup.

Alkaline Green Bean Casserole: Combine steamed green beans with a creamy sauce made from almond milk, nutritional yeast, and garlic. Sliced almonds are then sprinkled on top.

Alkaline Stuffing: To prepare an alkaline stuffing, combine sprouted grain bread with sautéed onions, celery, and herbs like sage and thyme.

Alkaline Roasted Brussels Sprouts: For a tasty and nutritious side dish, roast Brussels sprouts with olive oil and balsamic vinegar.

Alkaline Roasted Butternut Squash Soup: For a soothing soup, roast butternut squash with garlic and onion before blending with almond milk and spices.

Quinoa and pomegranate salad that is alkaline is produced by combining cooked quinoa with chopped herbs, pomegranate seeds, and a lemon-olive oil vinaigrette.

Alkaline Roasted Beet Salad: Toss mixed greens, walnuts, and an apple cider vinegar and Dijon mustard dressing with roasted beet slices after they are tender.

Sliced apples with cinnamon sprinkled on them are baked till tender and served as a wholesome treat.

Alkaline Gingerbread Cookies: To create a healthier version of gingerbread cookies that are still fun and tasty, use almond flour and coconut sugar.

Alkaline Chocolate Peppermint Bark: For a holiday treat, melt dark chocolate and whisk in peppermint flavor before topping with crushed candy canes.

Alkaline Spiced Hot Chocolate: For a cozy and warm Christmas beverage, reheat almond milk with cocoa powder, cinnamon, and nutmeg.

Alkaline Roasted Root Vegetables: For a tasty and wholesome side dish, roast a variety of root vegetables, such as carrots, parsnips, and turnips, with olive oil and herbs.

Alkaline Pecan Pie: To make a healthier version of pecan pie that is still decadent and delicious, combine maple syrup with almond flour.

The pleasures and customs of the holiday season can still be enjoyed while adhering to a healthy, balanced diet with the help of these alkaline holiday dishes. Include these recipes on your Christmas dinner for a delightful spread that is both healthful and filling.

ENTERTAINING WITH AN ALKALINE DIET

An alkaline diet may make entertaining delicious and healthful. To help you throw a successful celebration, here are some advice and recipes:

Serve alkaline water: Set up a station where attendees may hydrate throughout the event with alkaline water and fresh fruit slices.

Alkaline components can be used to make tasty dips like guacamole, which is created with avocado and lime juice, or hummus, which is produced with chickpeas and tahini.

Provide platters of fresh veggies: Arrange a selection of fresh vegetables, such as carrots, celery, bell peppers, and cucumbers, along with a delectable alkaline dip, such as a ranch dressing made with cashews or tahini.

Serve alkaline salads. A simple vinaigrette made with alkaline components like apple cider vinegar, lemon juice, and olive oil is ideal for a light and healthful alternative. Alkaline foods to include in a salad include mixed greens, avocado, and sprouts.

Alkaline proteins to grill include fish, chicken, and tofu that have been marinated in herbs and lemon juice.

Create alkaline desserts: Fruit salads with coconut whipped cream and energy balls composed of almonds, dates, and coconut flakes are two tasty and healthful raw vegan desserts.

Serve alkaline beverages: For a light and healthful beverage option, fresh juices made with alkaline elements like cucumber, celery, and lemon or herbal teas like chamomile or peppermint are ideal.

Make a charcuterie board that is alkaline: For a beautiful and healthy appetizer, arrange a variety of alkaline items like olives, roasted almonds, fresh fruit, and alkaline cheeses like goat or feta.

Provide alkaline mocktails, which are made by combining fresh fruit juice, sparkling water, and fresh herbs.

Create an alkaline dessert bar: For a tasty and nutritious dessert alternative, set up a dessert bar with raw vegan treats, fresh fruit, and toppings like coconut flakes and nut butter.

You may entertain with an alkaline diet and provide your guests with tasty, healthful options by adopting these suggestions and recipes.

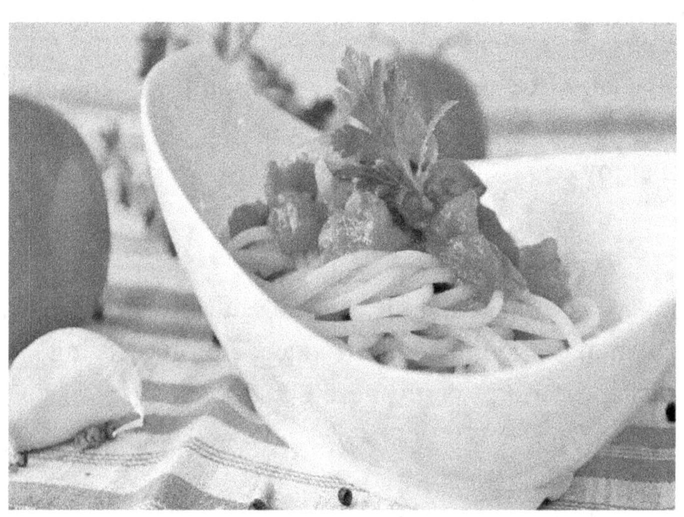

CHAPTER 10

ALKALINE DRINK RECIPES

The following recipes for alkaline drinks can be found in an acid-alkaline diet cookbook:

Ginger-Lemon Tea: Slices of fresh ginger, lemon juice, and boiling water should all be placed in a teapot. Strain after 5 to 10 minutes of steeping, then enjoy.

Sliced cucumber, mint leaves, and water should be combined in a large pitcher to make cucumber mint water. Before serving, let it steep for at least an hour in the refrigerator.

Blend 1 cup each of kale, spinach, banana, frozen mixed berries, 1 tablespoon of chia seeds, and 1 cup of coconut water to make an alkaline smoothie.

Blend 1 cup of frozen pineapple, 1 tablespoon of turmeric, 1 cup of almond milk, 1 tablespoon of honey, and a pinch of black pepper in a blender to make a pineapple-turmeric smoothie.

Juice one cucumber, one green apple, one lemon, one inch of ginger, and a handful of spinach to make a green juice.

Coconut Water Electrolyte Drink: Combine 1 cup coconut water, 1 tablespoon freshly squeezed lime juice, and a teaspoon of sea salt in a tall glass.

Juice 2 cups of watermelon, 1/4 cup of fresh mint leaves, and 1/4 cup of lime juice to make watermelon mint juice.

Hibiscus Iced Tea: In a teapot, combine boiling water, 2 to 3 hibiscus tea bags, and fresh ginger slices. Strain after 10-15 minutes of steeping, then serve over ice.

Green tea matcha latte: Heat 1 cup almond milk, 1 tablespoon honey, and 1 teaspoon matcha powder in a small pot. Stir until foamy and smooth.

Juice a few beets, an apple, a piece of ginger that is an inch long, and 1/4 cup of freshly squeezed lemon juice in a juicer.

Lemon Turmeric Water: Combine water, water, and 1/2 teaspoon of turmeric powder in a big glass. Stir well, then indulge.

Blend 1 cup of frozen blueberries, 1/2 cup of coconut milk, 1 banana, and 1 tablespoon of almond butter in a blender to make a blueberry smoothie.

Green Tea Ginger Lemonade: Combine 4 green tea bags, fresh ginger slices, 2 lemons' worth of juice, and 1 tablespoon of honey in a big pitcher. Strain after 10-15 minutes of steeping, then serve over ice.

Juice 1 orange, 1 carrot, and 1 inch of ginger in a juicer to make orange carrot juice.

Apple Cider Vinegar Tonic: Combine 1 tablespoon of apple cider vinegar, 1/2 a lemon's juice, 1 teaspoon of honey, and water in a big glass. Stir well, then indulge.

These recipes for alkaline drinks are healthy for the body and refreshing. They can assist the body replenish vital nutrients and strengthen the immune system while also enhancing digestion.

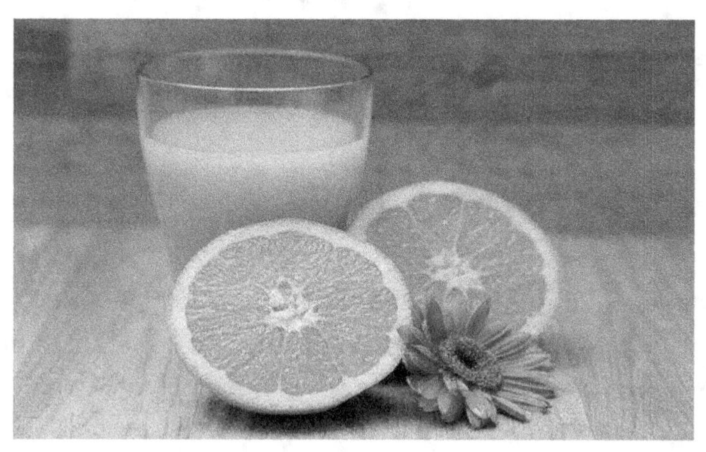

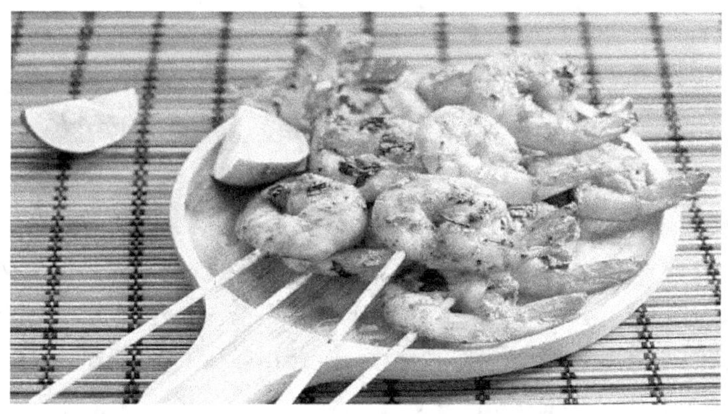

CHAPTER 11

SUPPLEMENTS AND VITAMINS FOR

AN ALKALINE DIET

Even while eating whole foods is usually optimal, it can occasionally be difficult to consume enough of some vitamins and minerals when following an alkaline diet. Supplements can be useful in certain situations to make sure the body receives what it needs. Consider these vitamins and supplements for an alkaline diet:

Multivitamin: Essential vitamins and minerals that may be missing from the diet can be provided by a high-quality multivitamin.

Vitamin B12: It can be difficult to get enough vitamin B12 on a plant-based, alkaline diet. Vitamin B12 is necessary for healthy neuron and red blood cells. Supplementing with vitamin B12 can assist to guarantee adequate levels.

Vitamin D: Vitamin D is necessary for strong bones, but getting enough from food alone might be difficult. Take into account increasing your sun exposure or taking a vitamin D supplement.

Magnesium: The diet frequently lacks magnesium, which is necessary for strong bones, muscles, and neurons. Magnesium levels can be made sufficient by taking a supplement.

Probiotics: Probiotics can assist maintain an alkaline diet by promoting good gut bacteria and enhancing digestion.

Omega-3 fatty acids: Omega-3s are crucial for brain and heart health, yet they are frequently missing in diets. Take into account taking an omega-3 dietary supplement, like fish oil or algae oil.

Zinc: Getting enough zinc from food alone can be difficult, yet it is necessary for a healthy immune system. If necessary, think about taking a zinc supplement.

An acid-alkaline diet, then, is a manner of eating that emphasizes ingesting foods that support balancing the body's pH levels. People can improve their general health and wellbeing by consuming a diet high in alkaline foods, such as fruits, vegetables, and plant-based proteins, while minimizing acidic items, such as processed meals, dairy products, and animal proteins.

In order to succeed on an acid-alkaline diet, keep in mind that you should prioritize whole, nutrient-dense meals and minimize processed and acidic ones. You may improve your overall wellness, have more energy, and enjoy improved health by including these dishes into your regular routine.

Before taking any supplements or vitamins, it's crucial to speak with a doctor to make sure they're safe and suitable for you. Furthermore, the main goal of an alkaline diet should always be obtaining nutrients from entire foods.

MOTIVATION TO MAINTAIN AN ALKALINE LIFESTYLE

Choosing to live an alkaline lifestyle can be difficult at first, but it is a choice that can improve your general health and wellbeing. It's crucial to maintain your motivation and support as you start to alter your food and lifestyle.

Here are several justifications for maintaining an alkaline diet and some advice for maintaining your motivation:

Increased Energy: Consuming an alkaline-rich diet will provide your body an increase in energy. Nutrient-dense alkaline foods can help control your blood sugar levels and prevent energy slumps throughout the day.

Better Digestion: Eating an alkaline diet can aid in digestion improvement and gas and bloating reduction. The fiber in fruits and vegetables can also aid in maintaining a healthy digestive system.

Weight control: An alkaline diet can support your efforts to keep a healthy weight. Alkaline foods are abundant in nutrients and low in calories, so you can feel filled without overeating.

A more alkaline diet can help strengthen your immune system. Leafy greens and other alkaline meals are abundant in antioxidants and other nutrients that can help shield your body from disease and illness.

Reduced Inflammation: Chronic disorders like arthritis and heart disease frequently result from inflammation in the body, which an alkaline diet can help to minimize.

Advice on How to Stay Motivated

Set attainable goals: Set attainable objectives and start small. Try not to make too many changes at once. Instead, start modest with your food and lifestyle improvements and gradually add more.

Connect with others who live an alkaline lifestyle to find support. Find a friend who is likewise interested in enhancing their health, or join an online support group.

Celebrate Your Successes — No Matter How Small — Celebrate Your Successes. Recognize your progress and use it as encouragement to keep going.

Concentrate on the Positive: Instead of concentrating on the foods you can eat on an alkaline diet, concentrate on how wonderful and nourishing they are.

Continue Learning: Keep abreast of the advantages of an alkaline lifestyle and continue picking up new cooking techniques and ideas for incorporating alkaline foods into your diet.

Finally, living an alkaline lifestyle can be a start in the right direction for improving your health and wellbeing. You may keep moving toward your objectives and reaping the many advantages of an alkaline diet by remaining inspired and motivated. Keep going forward and keep your attention on the constructive improvements you are making in your life because, as you know, minor changes may have a great impact.

30 DAYS ALKALINE DIET MEAL PLANNER

Day 1

Breakfast: Green smoothie made with spinach, kale, avocado, banana, and almond milk

Lunch: Quinoa salad with mixed greens, cherry tomatoes, cucumber, red onion, and lemon vinaigrette

Dinner: Grilled salmon with roasted asparagus and sweet potato wedges

Day 2

Breakfast: Chia seed pudding with fresh berries and sliced almonds

Lunch: Vegetable stir-fry with tofu, broccoli, bell pepper, mushrooms, and brown rice

Dinner: Lentil soup with a side salad of mixed greens and sliced cucumber

Day 3

Breakfast: Oatmeal with almond milk, sliced banana, and cinnamon

Lunch: Greek salad with mixed greens, cherry tomatoes, cucumber, red onion, feta cheese, and lemon vinaigrette

Dinner: Grilled chicken with roasted Brussels sprouts and brown rice

Day 4

Breakfast: Scrambled eggs with sautéed spinach and mushrooms

Lunch: Chickpea salad with mixed greens, cherry tomatoes, cucumber, red onion, and lemon vinaigrette

Dinner: Baked sweet potato with black beans, salsa, and avocado

Day 5

Breakfast: Avocado toast with sliced tomato and a drizzle of olive oil

Lunch: Grilled vegetable wrap with hummus, mixed greens, and sliced avocado

Dinner: Grilled shrimp with roasted zucchini and quinoa

Day 6

Breakfast: Greek yogurt with fresh berries and sliced almonds

Lunch: Lentil and vegetable soup with a side salad of mixed greens and sliced cucumber

Dinner: Grilled pork tenderloin with roasted carrots and brown rice

Day 7

Breakfast: Smoothie bowl made with frozen mixed berries, almond milk, and chia seeds

Lunch: Quinoa and vegetable stir-fry with tofu, broccoli, bell pepper, mushrooms, and brown rice

Dinner: Grilled beef steak with roasted asparagus and sweet potato wedges

Day 8

Breakfast: Omelette with sautéed mushrooms, bell pepper, and spinach

Lunch: Chickpea and vegetable stir-fry with brown rice

Dinner: Baked salmon with roasted Brussels sprouts and brown rice

Day 9

Breakfast: Green smoothie made with spinach, kale, avocado, banana, and almond milk

Lunch: Greek salad with mixed greens, cherry tomatoes, cucumber, red onion, feta cheese, and lemon vinaigrette

Dinner: Grilled chicken with roasted zucchini and quinoa

Day 10

Breakfast: Chia seed pudding with fresh berries and sliced almonds

Lunch: Lentil and vegetable soup with a side salad of mixed greens and sliced cucumber

Dinner: Baked sweet potato with black beans, salsa, and avocado

Day 11

Breakfast: Avocado toast with sliced tomato and a drizzle of olive oil

Lunch: Grilled vegetable wrap with hummus, mixed greens, and sliced avocado

Dinner: Grilled shrimp with roasted asparagus and sweet potato wedges

Day 12

Breakfast: Scrambled eggs with sautéed spinach and mushrooms

Lunch: Quinoa salad with mixed greens, cherry tomatoes, cucumber, red onion, and lemon vinaigrette

Dinner: Grilled pork tenderloin with roasted carrots and brown rice

Day 13

Breakfast: Greek yogurt with fresh berries and sliced almonds

Lunch: Vegetable stir-fry with tofu, broccoli, bell pepper, mushrooms, and brown rice

Dinner: Baked salmon with roasted zucchini and quinoa

Day 14

Breakfast - Quinoa porridge with almond milk, topped with berries and sliced almonds

Lunch - Grilled chicken breast with a mixed green salad (spinach, arugula, kale) and a lemon vinaigrette dressing

Dinner - Baked salmon with roasted vegetables (asparagus, zucchini, bell peppers)

Day 15

Breakfast - Avocado toast with sprouted grain bread and sliced tomatoes

Lunch - Chickpea salad with mixed greens, cucumber, and a lemon-tahini dressing

Dinner - Grilled sirloin steak with roasted sweet potatoes and steamed broccoli

Day 16

Breakfast - Blueberry smoothie bowl with spinach, banana, and chia seeds

Lunch - Lentil soup with a mixed green salad (romaine, cucumber, bell pepper) and a balsamic vinaigrette dressing

Dinner - Baked chicken thighs with roasted brussels sprouts and cauliflower

Day 17

Breakfast - Oatmeal with almond milk, topped with sliced bananas and walnuts

Lunch - Grilled portobello mushroom burger with sweet potato fries

Dinner - Baked cod with sautéed spinach and roasted beets

Day 18

Breakfast - Chia seed pudding with coconut milk, topped with sliced mango and shredded coconut

Lunch - Tuna salad with mixed greens, cherry tomatoes, and a lemon vinaigrette dressing

Dinner - Baked chicken breast with roasted root vegetables (carrots, parsnips, turnips)

Day 19

Breakfast - Scrambled eggs with sautéed spinach and mushrooms

Lunch - Roasted turkey breast with mixed greens, sliced apples, and a honey-mustard dressing

Dinner - Grilled shrimp with a mixed green salad (arugula, kale, spinach) and a lemon vinaigrette dressing

Day 20

Breakfast - Berry smoothie with almond milk and protein powder

Lunch - Vegetable stir-fry with tofu, broccoli, bell peppers, and brown rice

Dinner - Baked cod with roasted sweet potatoes and green beans

Day 21

Breakfast - Quinoa bowl with sliced avocado, cherry tomatoes, and a poached egg

Lunch - Grilled chicken breast with a mixed green salad (spinach, arugula, kale) and a lemon vinaigrette dressing

Dinner - Grilled sirloin steak with roasted vegetables (asparagus, zucchini, bell peppers)

Day 22

Breakfast - Green smoothie with kale, banana, and almond milk

Lunch - Lentil soup with a mixed green salad (romaine, cucumber, bell pepper) and a balsamic vinaigrette dressing

Dinner - Grilled salmon with roasted brussels sprouts and cauliflower

Day 23

Breakfast - Chia seed pudding with coconut milk, topped with sliced peaches and chopped almonds

Lunch - Chickpea salad with mixed greens, cucumber, and a lemon-tahini dressing

Dinner - Baked chicken thighs with roasted sweet potatoes and steamed broccoli

Day 24

Breakfast - Blueberry smoothie bowl with spinach, banana, and chia seeds

Lunch - Grilled portobello mushroom burger with a mixed green salad (romaine, cucumber, cherry tomatoes) and a balsamic vinaigrette dressing

Dinner - Baked cod with sautéed spinach and roasted beets

Day 25

Breakfast - Oatmeal with almond milk, topped with sliced bananas and walnuts

Lunch - Tuna salad with mixed greens, cherry tomatoes, and a lemon vinaigrette dressing

Dinner - Grilled shrimp with roasted root vegetables (carrots, parsnips, turnips)

Day 26

Breakfast - Scrambled eggs with sautéed spinach and mushrooms

Lunch - Roasted turkey breast with mixed greens, sliced apples, and a honey-mustard dressing

Dinner - Baked chicken breast with roasted sweet potatoes and green beans

Day 27

Breakfast - Berry smoothie with almond milk and protein powder

Lunch - Vegetable stir-fry with tofu, broccoli, bell peppers, and brown rice

Dinner - Grilled sirloin steak with a mixed green salad (arugula, kale, spinach) and a lemon vinaigrette dressing

Day 28

Breakfast - Quinoa porridge with almond milk, topped with berries and sliced almonds

Lunch - Grilled chicken breast with a mixed green salad (spinach, arugula, kale) and a lemon-tahini dressing

Dinner - Baked salmon with roasted vegetables (asparagus, zucchini, bell peppers)

Day 29

Breakfast - Avocado toast with sprouted grain bread and sliced tomatoes

Lunch - Chickpea salad with mixed greens, cucumber, and a lemon vinaigrette dressing

Dinner - Grilled chicken thighs with roasted root vegetables (carrots, parsnips, turnips)

Day 30

Breakfast - Quinoa porridge with almond milk, topped with berries and sliced almonds

Lunch - Grilled chicken breast with a mixed green salad (spinach, arugula, kale) and a lemon vinaigrette dressing

Dinner - Baked salmon with roasted vegetables (asparagus, zucchini, bell peppers)

Note: This meal plan includes a variety of nutrient-dense foods that are considered alkaline-forming, including vegetables, fruits, whole grains, and lean protein sources. It's important to note that while some foods may be considered alkaline-forming, the body maintains a delicate balance between acidity and alkalinity, and the alkaline diet has not been conclusively proven to have significant health benefits. As with any diet, it's important to consult with a Doctor before making significant changes to your eating habits.

BONUS

30 DAYS ALKALINE MEAL PLANNER JOURNAL

BREAKFAST	LUNCH	DINNER

MONDAY

BREAKFAST	LUNCH	DINNER

TUESDAY

BREAKFAST	LUNCH	DINNER

WEDNESDAY

<table>
<tr><td></td><td>BREAKFAST</td><td>LUNCH</td><td>DINNER</td></tr>
<tr><td>THURSDAY</td><td></td><td></td><td></td></tr>
</table>

<table>
<tr><td></td><td>BREAKFAST</td><td>LUNCH</td><td>DINNER</td></tr>
<tr><td>FRIDAY</td><td></td><td></td><td></td></tr>
</table>

<table>
<tr><td></td><td>BREAKFAST</td><td>LUNCH</td><td>DINNER</td></tr>
<tr><td>SATURDAY</td><td></td><td></td><td></td></tr>
</table>

BREAKFAST	LUNCH	DINNER
SUNDAY		

BREAKFAST	LUNCH	DINNER

MONDAY

BREAKFAST	LUNCH	DINNER

TUESDAY

BREAKFAST	LUNCH	DINNER

WEDNESDAY

BREAKFAST	LUNCH	DINNER

THURSDAY

BREAKFAST	LUNCH	DINNER

FRIDAY

BREAKFAST	LUNCH	DINNER

SATURDAY

SUNDAY

BREAKFAST	**LUNCH**	**DINNER**

MONDAY

BREAKFAST	**LUNCH**	**DINNER**

TUESDAY

BREAKFAST	**LUNCH**	**DINNER**

WEDNESDAY

BREAKFAST	LUNCH	DINNER

THURSDAY

BREAKFAST	LUNCH	DINNER

FRIDAY

BREAKFAST	LUNCH	DINNER

SATURDAY

	BREAKFAST	LUNCH	DINNER
SUNDAY			

BREAKFAST	LUNCH	DINNER

MONDAY

BREAKFAST	LUNCH	DINNER

TUESDAY

BREAKFAST	LUNCH	DINNER

WEDNES...

BREAKFAST	LUNCH	DINNER

THURSDAY

BREAKFAST	LUNCH	DINNER

FRIDAY

BREAKFAST	LUNCH	DINNER

SATURDAY

BREAKFAST	LUNCH	DINNER

SUNDAY

www.ingramcontent.com/pod-product-compliance
Lightning Source LLC
Chambersburg PA
CBHW061639250726
48659CB00004B/1304